TOURETTE WARRIORS

ISBN: 978-0-9989290-2-6

TOURETTE WARRIORS

INSPIRING STORIES OF RESILIENCE AND TRIUMPH

JASON MICHAELS

Let's Connect!

Thank you for your interest in my book! I'm thrilled that you are about to meet some extraordinary individuals through these pages. I hope their stories bless your life the way that they have blessed mine.

I would love to keep in touch with you. We can keep in touch through my monthly e-newsletter or through social media. These are the places that I update first with the latest news, speaking engagements, shows, book projects, and more. If we keep in touch, maybe we will get to meet in person someday.

To sign up for my monthly e-newsletter, please visit my website JasonMichaelsMagic.com.

My Socials Are…

- /jasonmichaelsmagic
- /jasonmichaelsmagic
- /jasonmichaelsmagic
- /in/jasonmichaelsmagic

DEDICATION

This book is dedicated to the Tourette Syndrome community. If you live with Tourette Syndrome, you are a warrior — someone I would define as having successfully engaged in a struggle or conflict. This title can also refer to someone who shows great vigor or courage. Having lived with Tourette Syndrome my entire life, that definition sounds like it perfectly describes those of us who have also managed to live a fulfilling life in spite of this neurological condition called Tourette's.

Unfortunately, you may have also had to put up with ignorance, bullying, and unfairness on a ridiculous level. You've probably had to learn how to advocate for yourself when you didn't want to. You've even had to stand up to powerful people and fight for your self-respect when it wasn't fair. To say that YOU ARE RESILIENT is an understatement.

As you read the following interviews, I think you will find that all of the people in this book have triumphed in their own way over Tourette's. Some have overcome traumatic childhoods while others fight to live the lives that they want on a daily basis. Warriors, truly.

I hope that as you read the stories each of these people has chosen to share, you will see a little bit of yourself in them. I also hope that you find yourself inspired by the grit and determination that these warriors bravely demonstrate daily.

When I was a teenager, living with Tourette Syndrome seemed almost impossible. I sometimes thought of it as my greatest weakness — or even a curse. I never could have imagined that years later I would view Tourette's as a gift, one that has allowed me to serve others.

Today you have a choice. You can weaken yourself by seeing the world through the lens of a victim of an uncontrollable, extremely challenging neurological disorder. Or, you can choose to see yourself as an empowered warrior who can live fearlessly and fight for what you believe in — no matter the circumstances. To say that perspective is important may be the most critical takeaway from this dedication.

I pray to God that you choose empowerment. Really, I do. No matter what you choose though, please know that you are welcome here.

Welcome to a community of strong, capable, courageous people - people just like you. Welcome to a community of warriors - Tourette Warriors, as I affectionately refer to us.

ACKNOWLEDGMENTS

First and foremost, thank you to God. I am who You say I am, a child of a loving Creator and a soul that is saved. I was given a second chance because I believe that Christ died on a cross and then arose from the dead to live again.

Thank You for creating and showing me a path that is uniquely mine. Thank You for teaching me faith. Thank You for guiding me in this incredible adventure. It hasn't always been easy, but it has always been worth it.

Thank you to my wife, Jacqueline. You showed me that someone outside of my immediate family could believe in my purpose and my vision. I was very skeptical of that for a long time. I am so very thankful for you, your support, and your love.

I would also like to acknowledge and thank everyone who has affirmed that my story of living with Tourette Syndrome spoke deeply to them. Hearing your comments and how you internalized the insights derived from my own experiences have pushed me through the path of resistance. You have helped me stay the course and believe that my message deserves to be heard.

Finally, I would like to thank each and every person who has shared their stories of living with Tourette's. If you agreed to be a part of this book, I cannot express my gratitude to you enough. With that said, even narratives that didn't make the final edit still matter. May God bless you and yours.

CONTENTS

INTRODUCTION

I was scrolling through Facebook one day and happened upon a group that I had previously joined for people with Tourette Syndrome and their loved ones.

A single post caught my attention which expressed the concerns of a mother whose daughter wanted to become a doctor. She was worried that her daughter's tics would prohibit her from fulfilling that dream.

While I could certainly empathize with what this mother was dealing with, I immediately thought to myself, "OMG, lady! It's disrespectful to ask a bunch of strangers for advice when they don't know your daughter or what she is capable of. That is her business."

I scrolled through the comments and was pleased to see that most people told her to be supportive of what her daughter wants to achieve in this blessing we call life. Unfortunately, as there are always naysayers, some people weighing in on the situation expressed doubt. That contradiction between optimism and overt negativity got me thinking, so I decided to scan the rest of the posts and see what people were discussing overall.

Numerous posts were from people newly diagnosed. Most questions pondered the reality of living a full existence with Tourette's. Understandably, many people wanted answers from those who had done this. It was the cliche "proof in the pudding" situation where they only felt like they could trust those who had also had to find their footing.

Questions ranged from topics like "What is it like to have a romantic relationship with someone that has Tourette's?" to "Is it possible to have what the masses would define as a successful career?" Others wanted to know the nitty gritty of what it was like to navigate every day with uncontrollable tics, twitches, and vocalizations.

The doubt and unease that these posts raised made me sad. You see, I occasionally wondered if I would be successful as a professional entertainer early on in my career because of the tough competition. Yet I never doubted myself due to Tourette's.

Sure, I've had to work hard my entire life to make a living as a magician and public speaker, but not because of the tics that come along with Tourette's. The hours I've clocked in are simply because success rarely comes as easy as we think it should. Becoming known in one's field takes far more work and effort than we realize early in a career.

While I had stronger self-belief than many of the people in this group, I could understand their fears on a rational level. Whether you're the one with Tourette's or the parent of a child with the diagnosis, there are often many more questions than answers. Particularly when you are in the middle of an intense period of tics, wondering if you can find someone to love and accept you is a very real worry. These are questions that you, Tourette Warrior, and your loved ones deserve honest answers to from people who have lived similar lives to yours.

To further my cause, I am guilty of being a champion and exuberant cheerleader for people who have chosen a non-traditional path. I get charged up when I talk to entrepreneurs, artists, and anyone else who is taking their future into their own hands because of their belief in themselves.

My desire to educate, inspire, and alleviate very real concerns is why I decided to write this book. I want to champion anyone living with Tourette Syndrome in hopes that they will understand they are capable of accomplishing anything they desire. I don't care if you want to have a traditional nine-to-five career or a non-traditional one, where the bills aren't necessarily guaranteed every month. If you are living with Tourette's and wondering if "normalcy" is in your future, I assure you that it is.

In these pages are interviews with people who are living with Tourette Syndrome while also living successful lives. They chose their paths and persevered until their desired accomplishments were realized.

The challenges of those of us with Tourette's may exceed the everyday difficulties that most people face; however, they don't have to define our journeys or prevent our success. I am here, as your Tourette's cheerleader, to stand in your corner and show through these pages that you can do anything you put your mind to. I hope you learn valuable lessons from the incredible people featured in these conversations.

CHAPTER 1

NIKKI BURDINE

JOURNALIST AND TELEVISION ANCHOR

Nikki Burdine is a two-time podcast host and the former co-anchor of Good Morning Nashville, a daily show that first brought her passion for storytelling to viewers across her home state of Tennessee.

Before joining WKRN, Nikki was a reporter and fill-in anchor at WUSA9 in Washington, D.C. Her career has also taken her to WLEX in Lexington, Kentucky; WHAG in Hagerstown, Maryland; and even the Washington Commanders.

Nikki remains loyal to her alma mater, The University of Tennessee, where she earned her bachelor's degree in journalism with an emphasis in political science. Throughout her career, she has been recognized with an Emmy Award and multiple Associated Press honors.

Prior to all her accomplishments, Nikki was diagnosed with Tourette Syndrome and had to learn how to control her tics to have a successful career in television, where you have to be poised, self-assured, and professional.

Jason Michaels: Nikki, as childhood is so important in terms of how we approach adulthood, what type of kid were you? Outgoing, introverted, curious?

Nikki Burdine: I've always been very outgoing. My nickname as a kid was "Showtime." I always wanted to be the center of attention and got in the habit early on of putting on plays, dance performances, and writing skits for my friends and family. I love being in front of people, which I think translated into my career as a reporter in adulthood.

Jason Michaels: Absolutely. When you were in school, did you study acting or any type of performance art formally?

Nikki Burdine: Oh, no. Everything was done intuitively. I would invite my neighbors over without telling my parents, and they would show up to our house just as I was putting on a play. I don't have any acting training at all because I never made it that far in terms of learning the craft. I was on the dance team, which was my preferred way of performing. I did whatever I could to be in front of people and at the center of the action.

Jason Michaels: That is funny because there are so many people I've talked to that have Tourette Syndrome and end up, for some mysterious reason, in either really creative endeavors or in front of audiences. When you're in a stressful situation, whether in front of the camera or in front of a group of people, are your tics suppressed?

Nikki Burdine: Yes. I'm always suppressing them, but I have found ways to get around releasing them so that my anxiety is quelled. In a way, I will do a mini version of the tic, if that makes sense.

Jason Michaels: Yeah. Do you sort of "mask" it? I hide my tics in other movements, such as moving my hands when I talk, so they look "normal."

Nikki Burdine: Yes. The tic that I am compelled to do is to scream and point and look up at the ceiling and blink a lot. But I can't do that when I'm reading the morning newscast. So, what I'll do instead is, I'll tap my finger on the desk, and I'll go something like this (Nikki clenched her jaw here) or go like this (she did a small tic here where it appeared as though she looked off to the side.) I'll also look up at the ceiling during commercial breaks, which allows me to give in to the tic a bit, or I'll clear my throat.

Every motion I've just described is normal and something most people wouldn't notice. But being able to release a mini-tic helps ease my anxieties so I can get through that moment. Then when I'm by myself, I can let all the tics out.

Jason Michaels: It's almost like when you have that commercial break, you're giving the Tourette's what it wants by letting out the tics. Then, you can get back to "normal." I get it completely. Do you recall the age you were when you started having tics?

Nikki Burdine: I was around twelve when I was diagnosed, although I'm sure it probably started before then. I have a terrible memory. My family always jokes that I don't remember anything; however, I believe it was a defense mechanism just to kind of block it out. I do recall it started around the time my dad was deployed to Desert Storm. A lot of people with Tourette's will say that their tics come on thanks to trauma, no matter how big or small, or a major life change. Looking back, I do believe my dad having to go overseas accelerated my tics coming out. My parents were like, "Whoa, whoa, whoa. What's going on?"

Jason Michaels: Speaking of that, did you feel like you had a strong support group at home?

Nikki Burdine: A thousand percent, which makes me feel very lucky. First of all, without my parents and my sisters, I do not think that I would be where I am today. Truthfully, I don't know if I would be alive. I definitely wouldn't be this successful, and I wouldn't be the type of person I am without them. They were so supportive, understanding, and helpful. My parents took this thing that nobody understood or knew anything about and said, "All right, we're going to figure this out. We're going to help her. We're going to get her what she needs and let Nikki be Nikki." They gave me the tools that I needed, without judgment, so I could be successful. My friend group was equally as amazing.

Jason Michaels: Did you experience any bullying moments?

Nikki Burdine: Again, with my memory being how it is, I think I kind of blocked them out. But I tell this story because I do have this one vivid memory. One of my tics, because as you know, they evolve, was to scream "papaya" when I was in middle school. So weird. After yelling that word, I would clamp my jaw really loud and then do the duck lip. Over and over my friends would be like, "What are you doing?" or "Why did that happen?" I became a spectacle that they wanted to watch because they thought it was funny. I'd be like, "Just do it. It's funny. Just do it."

Wanting to be the entertainer, provider of fun, and center of attention, I would do it because they asked me to. I have a picture of all my girlfriends in middle school in the early nineties making the now iconic duck face. I coped with Tourette's by making fun of my-self and the condition itself.

While bullying probably did exist, I was so protected by my family and friends that they sheltered me from it. In a way, I had the best situation possible.

Jason Michaels: Yeah, that's fantastic. I had a similarly supportive network of family members and find it unfortunate when people do not. Hopefully, they can find it in a peer group or somebody they can trust. What do you believe your level of severity was as far as your tics go? And did it change from childhood to adulthood?

Nikki Burdine: I would say when I was first diagnosed, the reaction to my tics was more so, "What is she doing? That's weird." Then they became very extreme. I would scream so loudly that my sisters would be like, "You're hurting my ears, Nikki. Mom, why is she doing this?"

It hampered my school experience because I would have to take tests by myself, which I oftentimes couldn't even finish. Math was a big source of anxiety for me and still is. I would write out my math problem, and then I would erase it. Repeatedly, I would do this again until I had a gigantic hole in my paperwork. Constantly scrubbing out the work I had just put down on paper was a tic that came on suddenly. Fortunately, my dad stepped in by rewriting my math problems so I wouldn't keep wiping out my homework.

Jason Michaels: Did a tic ever cause any serious harm to you or someone else physically?

Nikki Burdine: I totaled a car because I was ticking at one point.

Jason Michaels: Wow.

Nikki Burdine: While I don't remember which tic it was, one happened while I was driving. I slid off the side of the road, flipped the car, and ended up upside-down.

Jason Michaels: Oh my gosh.

Nikki Burdine: I even have a scratch on my forehead to this day. I'm so lucky nothing worse happened. So yeah, the tics burdened my daily life.

Jason Michaels: What was it like when you finally left the safety net of your house and went away to college?

Nikki Burdine: While I was medicated, the tics were still extremely rough during middle and high school. However, I was able to cope and clearly felt confident and supported enough to attend college. I went to the University of Tennessee.

The dramatic change of entering my freshman year of college sent my tics through the roof. I was on my own for the first time with no parental supervision or structure. Depression also kicked in then for the first time in my life. A general malaise combined with anxiety and my tics were kind of the perfect storm. When I became a freshman, things got really dark and my tics worsened. I became suicidal.

Jason Michaels: What were some of the behaviors you were exhibiting at the time that made it clear you were depressed?

Nikki Burdine: So, I was on all this medication, and I wasn't getting out of bed. My roommates were like, "What's going on? We're worried about Nikki. We know something's not right."

I wasn't going to class, and I hadn't gotten out of bed in two weeks. Finally, my mom drove to campus, took me to the doctor, and I was prescribed a handful of pills. I probably took about nineteen pills at a time, twice a day, as a kid still in my teens.

Jason Michaels: Did this help or was it still very much the same?

Nikki Burdine: I wasn't suicidal anymore. While my tics were better, I was an absolute zombie. I also put on thirty pounds in a month, and my mom finally said, "All right, this is not good. Our daughter's alive, but this isn't Nikki. She's a shell of herself, and this is not a way forward for her to live." So, my mom did all kinds of research and got me down to one medication, Zoloft, which I've been on ever since. Yet the real turning point was tuning out all the outside noise and focusing on the root cause of my anxiety and depression. In turn, that self-work helped me to manage my tics. While I still have them, along with occasional bouts of anxiety and depression, all of it is manageable. I attribute being able to overcome this dark period in my life to my mom.

Jason Michaels: What I'm hearing you say is that a support group is a big deal when it comes to living with Tourette's.

Nikki Burdine: A strong support network has been everything to my journey of healing, going all the way back to middle school. Had it not been for my friends, parents, sisters, or even my college roommates who said, "Hey, call her mom because something isn't right," I wouldn't be where I am today. Even the empathy people showed when I was crying on the floor or lying like a vegetable in my bed all contributed to a more positive outcome.

Jason Michaels: As an adult, I guess you're in a different situation with a different support group.

Nikki Burdine: I have an understanding with my friends and family that "Nikki's doing" whatever she's doing. If it is something weird, they just ignore it. The same goes with my colleagues at work.

I used to never talk about Tourette's at work. While I wasn't ashamed of it, I didn't want to be treated differently. Now it's almost like a point of pride that I accomplished all these things in spite of having Tourette's. It's like I think, "Oh, yeah. I also have these tics."

Jason Michaels: When I speak to groups, I say, "I'm going to tell you something that might sound crazy. Sometimes the things that we struggle with the most today, we might look at tomorrow and realize, in a weird sort of way, were a gift." You can objectively actually look at it and say, "I wouldn't be who I am today without this barrier I've overcome." So yeah, I totally get it. Have your tics ever stopped you from getting something you badly wanted?

Nikki Burdine: If it did, I didn't know it. While I certainly haven't been hired at every position I wanted, I got everything that was meant for me. Tourette's definitely didn't hold me back. Or, at the very least, if an opportunity didn't pan out due to my condition, I wasn't aware of it. But I still don't think that's the case.

Jason Michaels: You sound totally comfortable talking about it. How early on in a relationship do you feel comfortable talking about Tourette's?

Nikki Burdine: While I am very much at ease talking about Tourette's, I don't lead with it as a conversation starter. It's never "Hi, I'm Nikki and I have Tourette's." But if the opportunity arises, as in somebody mentions Tourette's or mental health, I volunteer my own experience right up front. Their first reaction is usually, "What? Really? I had no idea." I see this as my moment to be like, "This is what it's all about," especially because people are usually shocked when they find out. This is especially true on social media because, by looking at a photo of me, you would have no idea that I suffer from Tourette's. But like you, I really wasn't comfortable talking about it openly until my mid-to-late twenties.

Jason Michaels: What changed?

Nikki Burdine: Encouragement from friends, as their reaction was generally positive. To hear even strangers say, "Wow, that's incredible" made me start to look at it differently. I started viewing Tourette's as something that actually made me more special. It went from feeling sorry for myself to "Look what I've been able to accomplish, especially with a disability on top of it." It made me respect myself and others more and see us as the bad-asses that we are. "I should brag about this a little more" is what I started to think, which was a total change of tune.

That mind switch changed. Then I also started to hear from people when I would open up about it: "My son has Tourette's." Or someone's grandson or granddaughter who I happened to cross paths with had it. People asking if they could give their loved ones my phone number felt amazing. It also led to me forming connections with mothers who were worried about their kids. I am honest with these parents, who see me as an example of strength, that my tics were debilitating. They have absolutely impacted my life and I hope to always make that clear. However, I also let them know that I have still been able to accomplish everything I wanted to. Hopefully, it is encouraging for parents to see an example of someone that overcame Tourette's. I am happy to serve as some semblance of hope.

Jason Michaels: Did you also find that speaking about Tourette's was a way to normalize it? In my own experience, being open made me less embarrassed. I started to see this condition as simply an extension of myself.

Nikki Burdine: Oh my gosh, I used to be embarrassed for sure to the point that I would never talk about it. Absolutely no way, no how. Yet I also think the way the world is evolving, everything is more acceptable. That mentality has made having Tourette's a lot easier, whereas when we were kids, you didn't talk about your feelings — let alone a medical disorder. Tourette's would be like the lowest topic of conversation on the totem pole because it's not considered cool, you know?

Jason Michaels: I always felt like, "And on top of it, you have the weirdest medical condition of them all." While Tourette's is certainly serious, I like to hear about the lighter side of it. Are there any funny stories or situations you can recall that happened because of your Tourette's? I'm thinking of one where looking back you can say, "Wow, that's pretty hilarious actually."

Nikki Burdine: One of my two younger sisters tells this story best. We were in high school; I'm aged fifteen and she is thirteen, and both in that awkward, difficult stage of life. And while I don't remember this, she says that I would be up in my room doing my tics, which was screaming at the very top of my lungs. When her friends would be over and, naturally, ask, "Is that your sister screaming up there?" she would lie and say, "No, that's our cat." (Laughs) That's how high-pitched I was. It's still our inside-joke today.

Jason Michaels: Oh my goodness! It sounds like you would look at Tourette's, at this point in your life, and say, "This condition has made me a stronger and more empowered person." Has it helped you to look at situations that others might find challenging with a different, more solution-oriented point of view?

Nikki Burdine: For sure, however in middle and high school I would have had a dramatically different answer for you. I hated having Tourette's.

Jason Michaels: Of course. That point of view only seems natural for a child or teenager.

Nikki Burdine: It made everything more difficult, and I wanted nothing more than just to be normal. But once I got through that dark period of my freshman year of college and progressed into my sophomore year, it was like I found my passion. I found what I wanted to do with my life, and it was like nothing could stop me. In fact, Tourette's only heightened my work ethic and caused me to become even more focused. In a way, having a barrier made me even more successful.

Jason Michaels: Can you speak to passion a little more at length? Many people I've interviewed for this book have explained how important it is to find something you can invest in.

Nikki Burdine: Every time I speak to a mother who's worried about their child, my first instinct it to ask, "What does your child enjoy doing?" And they say, "Oh my gosh, they are obsessed with gymnastics," or "Soccer is their favorite way to spend an afternoon." My advice is for them to lean into that passion and enroll the child in as many lessons as they can. When I was in high school, I danced competitively. My parents would always say, "How in the world can you do this routine for three and a half minutes flawlessly without ticking at all? But then you sit at the dinner table, and you can't get through a conversation." And I never had an answer for it.

Jason Michaels: When I'm on stage, the exact same thing happens to me. I've never had an answer for why it happens, other than I think it is a God-thing.

Nikki Burdine: I think every person who has Tourette's can say the same thing. When your mind is that focused, we know if we break for a single second then a waterfall of tics might come on. We won't recover from that dramatic shift for a while. So, it's focus, focus, focus until we get through that moment, whatever it is. For me, it was a dance routine.

And then when I went to college, I was like, "What do I want to do with my life?" And television journalism was it for me. And once again, the first thought that goes through people's minds is, "How can you be a TV news anchor with Tourette's? Aren't you just going to scream out four letter words all the time?" And I say, "Of course not. Not every person who has Tourette's is afflicted the same way. Also, that's not all we do." I feel fortunate that I am able to hone in on the present moment, whether it was a dance routine or delivering current events.

Now, don't get me wrong, because during the commercial break, most likely in the bathroom, I'm going to do some weird things. Nevertheless, finding out what your passion is and focusing on that is the best way to control your tics. You may really love math, battling on the debate team, or enjoy reading. No matter the pursuit, find that and go in one hundred percent. Every person I've ever met with Tourette's has something that they really love or excel at.

Jason Michaels: Yes. A hundred percent. That's great. Did you have any techniques that you used to hide or mask any of the tics when you were younger? I looked at it as totally embarrassing. Was there anything that you did to help with the humiliation factor?

Nikki Burdine: Yes. A couple of things. One, I would say going back to the picture of my girlfriends, making the duck face and embracing rather than fighting my tic so that it became "a thing" rather than something to hide.

Jason Michaels: Oh, you mean highlight it.

Nikki Burdine: Yes, in a way I made it a quirky personality trait. Now that's not the case for every tic. Some of my screaming tics, that's not quirky or cute. So, to get around that, I would make sure that my teachers knew I had Tourette's. If I needed to be excused to go to the bathroom to scream at the top of my lungs, that's what I did. I wasn't being a delinquent student. I wasn't trying to skip class. However, having an open dialogue with my parents and teachers

Finally, there is behavioral therapy. Right now, I'm having this conversation with you, but what I really want to do is a big tic. Instead of doing that, I'm going to do something small where you may not even notice it, but it helps me get through this conversation.

Jason Michaels: Right.

Nikki Burdine: Evolving throughout my entire life has helped me.

Jason Michaels: Were your teachers receptive to the information you gave them like that you might need to scream in the bathroom from time to time? Also, I would be curious to know if your parents advocated for you ahead of those conversations.

Nikki Burdine: Most were supportive; however, the smartest move my parents made was setting up meetings with all of my teachers once I was diagnosed. Some were with me and other meetings were solo. That transparency set me up for success. The general theme of the conversations was, "Look this is what's going on. Nikki is not a bad kid, and there is a reason for her behavior. She's not trying to be disruptive."

Most of the teachers were like, "Okay, we got it. We will work together with you on this." That is except for my math teacher,

Mr. Trent, who I will never forget. In either sixth or seventh grade, he would accuse me of cheating on my math homework because my dad had to help me with it. Thankfully, my parents went in and set up a conference where they explained, "Look she has this tic where she erases her homework over and over. Therefore, her father has to help her with it. Here is a letter from her doctor explaining the diagnosis."

Even after seeing the medical paperwork, he still accused them of lying and never came around to accepting my condition. He was convinced that we were making Tourette's up; that it wasn't a real thing. That made math class, which was already difficult for me, ten times more stressful a situation. Of course, the anxiety made the tics ten times worse. It still amazes me how one horrible teacher could affect me my entire life. When I took my math placement exam in college, I had what I now perceive as a panic attack and tested into the absolute lowest level. I believe it was Math 100 or something embarrassingly low.

Jason Michaels: Stress, as you said, exacerbates the tics making them even worse. So, what would you want a parent or friend of someone with Tourette's to know? While it is kind to say you want to be supportive, if you haven't lived through the condition, it's hard to know what it's like.

Nikki Burdine: Advice should vary based on the person's age and their personality. When I was in middle school, my parents' first instinct was to put me in therapy, which I hated. I did not want to talk about Tourette's. Rather, I wanted to bury this thing under the rug and not look it in the eye.

If you have a kid like that, one who does not want to face this challenge head on, just be there to support them and listen when they are ready to talk. Forcing me to open up about it would never make that happen. My parents gave me a safe space to tic out whenever I needed to without giving it unnecessary attention.

As strange as it might sound, I wanted to tic alone. Coping with my tics solo allowed me to get it all out of my system. The last thing I wanted was not attention, but rather to get that energy out so I could move on with our conversation or the action I was doing.

Some kids might feel differently, which could lead to a conversation where you say, “Hey, listen, when you have these tics, what do you want me to do? Do you want me to ignore you? Do you want me to walk away? Do you want me to pretend like it's not happening?” That's what I wanted, but every kid might be different.

As an adult, I still very much want that; to be left alone to do my thing. As long as I’m not bothering you, there is no need to talk about it. If I want to, I will.

Jason Michaels: If you were speaking to someone who had just been diagnosed with Tourette’s, what would you say to them in regard to their future? How would you encourage them? Or what would you say their future looks like?

Nikki Burdine: The first piece of advice I would give is to find a support group of other people your own age with Tourette’s. The most important thing is to find somebody that you can talk to. If you are open to therapy, it can help you make it through the day. I think therapy can really help with finding the right behavior mechanisms. Finally, if you want to do your tic, find one that helps quell your anxiety and a safe space where you can release it.

Jason Michaels: Any other words of wisdom?

Nikki Burdine: If you're comfortable doing so, talk to your employer about it and say, “Look, if you notice me doing these weird things, this is what's up. I'm not on drugs. I'm not drunk at work. It's an official diagnosis." Also make sure that you take time for your mental health, because so many of us with Tourette's also have anxiety and depression along with other mood disorders. Personally, when my anxiety and my depression are under control, then my tics are way better.

Jason Michaels: Tell me a little bit about your career and some of the cool things you've accomplished. I want to know how you've gone from a twelve year old with Tourette's to being a star. You're on the news and on many people's televisions on a daily basis. So give me some highlights that you're particularly proud of.

Nikki Burdine: When I was in college, I knew I wanted to be in TV news, but I didn't really want to go straight to a small market. You're probably familiar with this story, which is that news anchors must start in a small town — or at least this was the way when I was a newbie. Instead, I rebelled and moved to DC and worked for the Washington Football Club, where I did marketing, even though I knew it wasn't the right career for me.

Then I said, "Okay, maybe I do need to go live in this small town, work this job, and do the grunt work as lowest man of the totem pole reporter." My first job was in Hagerstown, Maryland, which is an hour outside of DC and I was there for three years. Then I got a job in Lexington, Kentucky anchoring the weekend show. From there, my goal began to crystallize. I wanted to be a reporter in DC because I loved politics and everything about Capitol Hill, which I consider our nation's heartbeat. I always wanted to do that, so I got a job working for the CBS station as a reporter.

I lived in DC for five years or so — completely focused on my initial goal — which was to go to network and work for CNN, Fox News, or ABC. New York City was always the end goal because that was where I believed the premium anchor jobs were.

However, as they sometimes do, my plans changed dramatically for the better. My husband and I had just gotten back from a wedding in Nashville, where my agent had set up a meeting with the news director at a station. Immediately after that meeting, they offered me the job, and I told my husband, "I want to chase my dream of going to network." Still, I thought I had to be in a large market to pursue this. Instead, he played the devil's advocate and said, "That's fine. I'll support you, but you were so happy in Nashville. That's where all your people are, so really think about it."

Low and behold, he was right. After I accepted the job, I quickly got promoted to "Good Morning Nashville," which was realizing my dream of anchoring a show. It was all mine. Plus, I love mornings and felt that on this particular show I could have some fun and let my personality shine. Even though I didn't go the traditional network route, I feel as though I accomplished everything I set out to. Plus, on top of it, I became a mom. "Good Morning Nashville" was a show that allowed me to have a fulfilling home life and not have to chase tornadoes or shootings while looking after my child. Every choice I had made led me down the most perfect path.

As far as large accomplishments go, I would say covering a White House press briefing is pretty cool. Getting to interview President Biden, who was the Vice President at the time, was also exciting. Covering inaugurations, going live right in front of the iconic White House, winning my first Emmy, and talking to people whom I would have otherwise never met. Visiting the hollers of Eastern Kentucky and telling the stories of rural folks who nobody had previously listened to was particularly meaningful. It meant that they trusted me to relay their voice. Truthfully, it's all been pretty special.

Jason Michaels: I would say so. Through hard work, drive, and not taking "no" for an answer you've done so much. It would have been so much easier for you to view yourself as a victim and let Tourette syndrome hinder the potential you had.

Nikki Burdine: I think if anything, it propelled me.

Jason Michaels: That's fantastic. Just thinking about who might pick up this book, from a parent to an adult who was diagnosed later in life, is there anything else you want to share? Maybe they grew up in a small town, and then years later they found out they had Tourette syndrome. Is there anything that you want to share outside of what you've already shared? I'm very appreciative of the incredible value you've already added to this conversation.

Nikki Burdine: Doctors and medication can be wonderfully helpful. However, if you are someone that has Tourette's, always trust your gut. Similarly, for mothers reading this, listen to your intuition. While medical professionals do their best, they don't know your child like you do. If my mother had listened to those doctors who had me on nineteen pills twice a day, who knows where I would be? She knew that something was wrong and took matters into her own hands, which in turn saved my life. If something feels off, figure it out. Trust your own intuition because, like my own mother's, it's probably right on.

JASON'S SUMMARY

Nikki's story is a powerful reminder of how important a support group is when it comes to coping healthfully with Tourette's. Fortunately for her, Nikki's parents were in tune with their daughter and ready to step in when she needed their help. They advocated for her when she was dealing with difficult situations.

I find it refreshing that Nikki was able to count on her friends to embrace the tics that she experienced as opposed to making fun of her for doing something "off." She was even able to turn her tics into bonding experiences by encouraging her friends to have fun and emulate them.

As a young adult, Nikki overcame the embarrassment that tics often create by embracing herself. I wasn't as fortunate as Nikki to have friends who encouraged me early on. However, I finally found the courage in my thirties to talk about my own experiences with Tourette Syndrome tics thanks to Stephen Bargatze, a close friend.

I couldn't agree more with Nikki's advice to find a support group filled with other people who have successfully navigated Tourette's. In my program on resiliency, one of my key points is to find someone who you trust that you can talk to. Talking honestly and openly about having Tourette's helped me normalize it in my own life. That was a major accomplishment for me. With that said, Nikki is 100% correct that it might take others more time to open up about their feelings. To alleviate the pressure for anyone who is reading this, it took me until I was an adult to get there.

When Nikki spoke to embracing your passion, I felt like she was preaching to the choir. After speaking to many people with Tourette Syndrome, and living with it myself, it has become increasingly obvious that this population finds a source of fulfillment and dives wholeheartedly into it. Similar to those with ADHD, we often have incredible hyper-focus that leads to doing what we love at a very high level. That, in and of itself, is quite a superpower.

The final thing I wanted to bring up is behavioral therapy which Nikki addressed when she said, "Right now I'm having this conversation with you, but what I really want to do is a big tic. Instead of doing that, I'm going to do something small where you may not even notice it, but it helps me get through this conversation."

This type of coping mechanism has worked for me as well. Comprehensive Behavior Intervention for TICS (CBIT) is a type of therapy that can be transformative. It acknowledges the tic by teaching the person how to do a smaller one, which helps them manage their lives more effectively. By "paying the piper," those of us who live with tics can indulge in this urge while avoiding more disruptive and chaotic moments. While this isn't a perfect solution, it has been effective for many of us, me included.

To watch the video of the full interview with Nikki Burdine, access additional tools to help you live and thrive with Tourette Syndrome, and connect with the Tourette Warrior community, please visit TouretteWarrior.com.

In the next chapter, the interview with Heather Ramsey, Heather discusses her experience with CBIT. She also shares some incredible stories of how she educates and advocates for people with Tourette Syndrome in schools and with police officers and first responders.

CHAPTER 2

HEATHER RAMSEY

CO-FOUNDER GREATER CAROLINAS TOURETTE GROUP

Heather Ramsey is the Director of the Greater Carolinas Tourette Group. She educates and advocates for people living with Tourette Syndrome in her community and several states. Heather is an incredible example of someone who walks the walk and talks the talk. Her interview should be required reading for teachers, police officers, and anyone who wants to help people in positions of authority better work with those of us with Tourette's.

Heather Ramsey: I am the co-founder and leader of the Greater Carolinas Tourette Group which I started in 2014 because there is very little support in North or South Carolina. While I live in North Carolina, I was raised in South Carolina where, many years later, I still recognize the disparity. Both my kids have Tourette Syndrome, as do I, however, I didn't receive my diagnosis until my son did. While this might sound shocking, I was part of that fifty percent that go undiagnosed.

Yet I did get diagnosed when I was a child by a doctor who told my mom, "Well, Tourette Syndrome." Her response was, "Oh no, we're fine. It's not that. We're good." And move along.

So, I understand the stigma associated with it because of how my own family was in denial around my initial diagnosis. When the doctor was explaining my son's diagnosis, she said, "So it's hereditary. He got it from you, Heather." My husband looks at me quizzically, and naturally I say, "Back up a second." Her response was "Have you never received a proper diagnosis?" The look on my face must have said it all because she said, "Well now you have."

So that was a really big shock. Plus, on top of dealing with my own diagnosis, I was also grappling with my son's diagnosis. Probably much in the same vein as my mother grappled with questions around my diagnosis, I also wondered, "How do I empower him? Or, do we just ignore this? Should we confide in friends and family? What's the best way to go about all of this?"

My husband is a very reserved and private person, who tips farther on the introverted scale than me. He said, "I don't think we need to tell anybody." When I started thinking about it, I thought: ***what message is that sending? If we are telling our son to fake it or suppress it, what kind of message is that sending?***

I remember growing up and getting bullied for my behaviors, so I figured out ways to hide Tourette Syndrome. That's what I did when I was younger, and while it is how I adapted to my surroundings, it wasn't fun.

Clearly, I wasn't successfully hiding my tics because the doctor saw them like a glaring red stoplight. So, I decided embracing my condition was the best approach because, if I couldn't accept myself, then how could I empower my son to do the same? I feared if we conveyed the message that we were ashamed of his condition, then it would just perpetuate the stigma that's associated with Tourette Syndrome.

One thing I tell people is you can try to hide Tourette's, but you won't be very effective at camouflaging it. Also, what kind of life is that to be inauthentic all of the time? Having lived that myself I knew it wasn't the best approach for my son.

He graduates college a week from today, a huge accomplishment for anyone, let alone someone with Tourette's. There were many times in elementary, middle, high school, I wondered, "How is this going to pan out?" With all the co-occurring conditions and the executive dysfunction that goes along with it, I really worried about his future. From all the struggles he had in school to now, that college degree is a culmination of his effort and drive. This achievement is all him, and I'm very happy for the hurdles he's overcome.

Jason Michaels: Your perspective is fascinating because of the diagnosis you received at that first doctor's appointment. As a grown adult, you're having to process the shock of being misinformed as a child and probably thinking ***how do I move forward from here?***

Heather Ramsey: I tell my son frequently, "If I knew then what I know now, I would've done so many things differently." I relate this to life in general, but particularly with school.

Now I know about best practices and educational accommodations that can be made to support a student with Tourette's. On one hand, I feel incredibly guilty for not being better equipped to deal with my son. I was doing the best I could at the time, and I'm just grateful he's resilient.

My daughter was diagnosed two years later. So, my husband feels very much out of the loop here. It's a house full of Tourette Syndrome.

Naturally with the knowledge I have now, I know I would have been able to create a better situation for both my kids back then. The benefit of education and training around Tourette's is that I can help people now with the acumen I've gained the way I wish I could have then.

There are so many trying situations, which oftentimes feel violating, that people with Tourette's deal with on a daily basis. If I can reduce even a portion of them, I'll consider myself victorious.

School is the biggest obstacle because Tourette's still isn't a household word in many places. There is shame and stigma and the "sweep it under the rug" mindset. Thanks to the negligence of education, parents and other adults must lean on one another for support in terms of how to inform.

Then there comes the question: How do you treat it? There isn't one tried and true methodology. So, there are just a lot of obstacles that people with Tourette's have to overcome, and school should not be one of those. I really believe that.

I sincerely believe knowledge creates tolerance, and therefore acceptance, which is why I work with schools to educate them about Tourette's. Everybody is irritating in one way or another. If there was more knowledge around Tourette Syndrome and the odd behaviors that come along with it, maybe people would be a little less judgmental. People may throw stones, but they shouldn't because of the flaws behind their own glass houses.

Jason Michaels: Let's say you're a parent, and you want to talk to your child's teachers about their behavioral quirks, what is the best way to go about doing that?

Heather Ramsey: Meeting your child's teachers in person at the beginning of the school year will make the biggest difference. Only then will you be able to gauge their response in reaction to your child's diagnosis. The teachers will also be familiar with the condition and know what to expect. I'll never forget the day I told one of my son's teachers that he had Tourette Syndrome. As we walked through the halls, she turned around shaking her head and saying, "No, he doesn't. That's not a thing." And I sarcastically snapped back, "Okay. Well, I didn't realize you had your MD."

As odd as it may seem, I also tell every teacher to ignore the behavior.

When I do in-service training for teachers, they'll often ask, "But if somebody is yelling, 'Fuck you', what am I supposed to do?"

And I tell them, "You're the adult, and your students will follow your lead." Their next question is naturally about HIPPA and a fear around disclosing the child's identity or medical condition. My response is, "Tourette Syndrome kind of outs itself."

While it might sound extreme, having a routine educational talk every year for five minutes at the beginning of each class sets the tone for the year. As the tics come on, the teacher will feel more at ease ignoring them so that the behavior becomes almost background noise, a non-issue. The teachers who are ill-informed and lack a plan struggle with what to do when that situation arises. That's when things get out of hand.

Jason Michaels: Have you ever had to revisit a situation and re-educate a teacher or advocate more vehemently for the child's rights?

Heather Ramsey: Yes, a hundred percent, ironically last month. It is heartbreaking to see what this young man has endured. He's at a charter school in North Carolina, [which] I have had a lot of struggles educating. While you can provide the learning materials, you can't make someone comprehend it.

I've seen both sides of the coin. The more favorable one is obviously when you see the light bulb moment behind a teacher's eyes or in their facial expression. That is when you know your instruction has catalyzed an 'aha' moment — they get it. Then I have also done trainings where I've wondered if the teachers were even in attendance because of how little they got out of the seminar.

Jason Michaels: You're thinking, "Was this person in the same room as me?"

Heather Ramsey: Exactly right. I was stunned last month when I did an Individualized Education Program (IEP) at a school whose faculty was absolutely clueless about Tourette's. As I told the room filled with parents, students, and the special education team, "I am a Tourette resource with X number of years' experience training schools and individual families on how to handle Tourette's." It was clear if they weren't sure what to do, they could ask me. I'm not an advocate for any particular student or school but rather, stand for Tourette Syndrome.

At the end of the meeting, I felt great about the way things had gone in respect that everyone was grateful to get started. They said, "We will definitely get training scheduled for all the teachers, and thank you for your wealth of knowledge." From there, we started pulling together the accommodations.

A few weeks later, I drove two and a half hours to give the training and was blown away by the questions, comments, and feedback. All revolved around how they could punish and discipline people afflicted by Tourette's.

Jason Michaels: Were you appalled hearing this? If so, I would say that.

Heather Ramsey: I was like, "What?" And then one person said, "So what I'm hearing is we can never punish someone with Tourette Syndrome?" No, I unequivocally never said that. I'm saying you should not punish a disability. The whole point of punishment and discipline is to change behavior which is impossible with Tourette's because it is an inherent condition. Lastly, a teacher is there to provide support, rather than manage Tourette Syndrome which is the responsibility of the individual and their families. That's simply not their role.

Jason Michaels: I've often thought, ***if I did not have Tourette Syndrome, it would be difficult to understand the uncontrollable nature of the tics.*** It almost sounds like this group of people that you were training didn't understand that tics truly are ungovernable.

Heather Ramsey: Exactly. In my two-hour training sessions, the first sixty minutes are the most critical because that is when I do a deep dive into the definition of an uncontrollable tic. If they say, "I don't understand how someone can't stop saying a word," I explain that there are no forewarnings. People do not know they will have a tic until it has happened. Therefore, you can't do much to prevent it. I would compare tics to breathing and blinking, which we oftentimes don't think much about.

Jason Michaels: Right. I understand how it would be hard for certain people to wrap their heads around that. Uncontrollable is easy to define and hard to fully comprehend.

Heather Ramsey: Correct. Even after breaking it down, most people still don't understand how someone could have zero control over their tics. Logically, I can empathize when I think of a young man I met years ago whose tic was to scream, "Fuck you!" and then fall on the ground. Even with as much knowledge as I have, I still found myself thinking, ***Can't you stop that?*** While his actions would technically fall under the gross motor skill category, that doesn't mean he had any control over it. And once you've broken the egg, it's shattered, which is frustrating.

Jason Michaels: Oh, incredibly frustrating. Just understanding what Tourette Syndrome entails is hard for some people to comprehend because it's so outside the norm.

Heather Ramsey: To relate to my audiences, I often use the reference of how wheelchairs made me uncomfortable as a child. I thought they were contagious. Therefore, it comes down to teachers setting the stage, particularly for small children, so they do not become unnerved around people that have Tourette's. I believe this comes down to familiarity through access to information and learning more about it.

And the federal government very clearly states, "We don't care if you feel uncomfortable, this is law around disabilities, and you must abide by it." I try to have a little more compassion for the teachers by saying, "I know this is difficult to deal with in a class of thirty or thirty-five; however, someone is going to walk in one day with Tourette's. It isn't a matter of if, but when. Therefore, I want to provide you with the armor and tools you'll need to maintain control of the classroom when they have an outburst." You will absolutely want to pull your hair out and can try to punish it, but I promise you that is going to damage the student further. Being shamed for their behavior will have a long-lasting effect on their psyche and self-esteem. Try to fight me on this, but you will lose because that is a fact.

Jason Michaels: And realistically, knowing how Tourette Syndrome works, isn't punishing it just going to exacerbate it?

Heather Ramsey: It absolutely does, which brings me to the culmination of what happened. The afternoon of my training, the student with Tourette's had an episode, and the staff didn't believe it was caused by a tic. Normally, I am reticent to give out my cell phone number because you can always reach me by email, but I had shared it with every teacher and administration member. I made it clear: "If a situation comes up, and you don't know what it is — before you act — call or text me. I will stop what I'm doing and help you get to the bottom of it, because that's how important it is to get this right."

They suspended the student and afterwards, they revoked his invitation to attend the school. Basically, it was an indefinite suspension. From there, a lawyer got involved. It was absolutely the most horrific thing I've ever experienced, and I was just an outsider, what I consider a Tourette resource. I can't imagine what that student and his parents had to endure with the school so blatantly ignoring the law and moralities in terms of what is right. At the end of the day, yes, it's law. In my eyes, either you do something because of integrity or the restrictions of the law. In spite of this, the school's attorney statement said, "We're not budging, and you can take us to court if you disagree." It's a shame because no family wants to go through a due hearing process, and neither does the government.

The most heartbreaking element was that his right to be a student was revoked because the institution refused to learn.

Jason Michaels: This just sounds like it's a school that said, "We don't care what the law is. You're not actually going to spend the money to take us to court. Even if you do, it'll take a year, and by that point in time, the problem is gone for us already." So, this is a situation where people in power abused their power, and it's just as simple as that.

Heather Ramsey: Yes.

Jason Michaels: While outrageous and infuriating, after reading a lot of different personal accounts, I have seen that it's more common than we realize for people with Tourette's to be treated poorly by others.

Heather Ramsey: You are exactly right, and it's a shame. I beat my head against the wall because, as I told these teachers, my goal was to help them. I did my best to empathize letting them know, "I can imagine your frustrations because you have no control. However, I can make your life easier and turn this whole ship around. Yet, this comes down to your perspective and being willing to change it." While I tried to explain that the child wasn't the problem, but rather had a problem, they refused to see it.

Jason Michaels: On a lighter note, tell me about some wins because I know you talk to teachers who do get it. I bet you have had plenty of experiences where you were able to enrich a student's life by helping their teachers better handle Tourette's.

Heather Ramsey: Yes, and those success stories are the reason I get up and pursue my line of work every day. They are why I keep plugging along and persisting through hard times. Also, as I explained before, if I had the acumen that I do now when my own children were growing up, they would have had a much more positive academic experience.

As a trainer who covers multiple states, I do both in-person and Zoom classes. One client with whom I had done in-person training, and then Zoom sessions, was still having difficulties and just not getting it. So, we set up an in-person training and after meeting with them face to face, I saw lightbulb moments. I mean, I literally saw their brains flashing because they were starting to see the disconnect. One teacher explained, "This one particular student reads his book all of the time which means he isn't paying attention" to which I explained, "That's an escape because he doesn't feel safe being himself. He intuitively knows that someone is going to fuss at him or start an issue." While it may not have been a physical safety issue, the bottom line was that he didn't feel at ease because there was always the threat of being harassed.

By retreating into his book, he found a space where he felt secure. I further related by telling them about my own son's perceived addiction to video games. My husband and I were pulling our hair out, too, until we found a therapist who explained, "The realm of video games is where your son feels accepted, liked for who he is, and free from ridicule." Finally, we realized that's his escape. That epiphany changed the way I saw my son's attraction to video games. While moderation is certainly important, my husband and I had gone about it the wrong way chastising him for this hobby. By looking at that outlet from a different perspective, we realized it was important to create more safe spaces so he didn't have to hide. In explaining this to the teachers they said, "We never thought about that. What is the next right move?" That's when I further explained that immense responsibility comes along with a 504 student*. Even if they have thirty-five students in their classroom that student with Tourette's, and co-occuring conditions, simply needs extra attention.

Teachers can alleviate their own frustrations by keeping a closer eye on the student, so they can prevent the antecedent that triggers tics. By explaining the importance of creating safe environments, the way teachers acquiesced was astonishing. I knew things were heading in the right direction when I received a call from a mother the next day saying, "Heather, the math teacher totally got it and like cold turkey, my son stopped reading as much in his classes." The change was drastic, and while a few teachers still didn't go along with the program, the bulk of them did. There will always be that one teacher who is stubborn, and you have to just accept it.

Administrators are another case, but those successes make the work worthwhile and are why I wake up wanting to fight every morning.

Jason Michaels: That's wonderful.

Heather Ramsey: The best-case scenarios are when the school nails it immediately. For example, I had a two-hour Zoom meeting with a school and family based in South Carolina. The school was already incredibly progressive in terms of the accommodations they were offering. One child was making such progress with occupational therapy that he could have easily been discharged. However, they chose to be proactive instead. "We're going to keep him on at thirty minutes a month," they explained, "because he is young and might need these strategies again to be successful in the future." My immediate reaction was, ***Why can't every school do that because their thoughtfulness made that family's life so much easier.*** That is the kind of mentality I wish for all schools.

Jason Michaels: Yeah, that's great.

Heather Ramsey: People in positions of power need to understand how to work with those of us with Tourette's. A recent win was receiving a grant from the Centers for Disease Control and Prevention (CDC) and Tourette Association to create an educational training video. The final product is a forty-plus minute overview of the condition and how law enforcement can facilitate smooth, positive encounters with anyone afflicted by it. One segment features a few of my Tourette youth ambassadors acting out a mock traffic stop with a local sheriff in the Carolinas. We felt this scenario would be relatable to officers. When you personalize an experience, even someone in a position of authority is willing to pay closer attention. The youth ambassadors were chosen strategically, like one who has coprolalia*. One of her tics is to, unfortunately, slap her dad in the face. I felt this was a relatable tic situation to demonstrate because it is one that an officer will likely come across. Our intention was to teach them how to respond appropriately, while also keeping themselves safe.

Another example we wanted to show is a business disturbance such as how a Walmart clerk can handle someone with coprolalia. Through acting out situations where the person says something offensive, shouts cuss words, or the police are called because items are knocked off the shelf due to an arm tic, law enforcement will know exactly what to do. This is especially important because police are obligated to tell management, "This is a covered disability, and the person has every right to be here. You cannot force them off the premises."

The last one we demonstrated is the domestic situation. This one is really interesting because in South Carolina, if you call 911 and say you have a domestic disturbance or domestic violence incident, the officers are required to make an arrest, which is scary. To further this point, Tourette rage is a real thing that deserves medical intervention. When a dad encounters a violent situation, he might call the police and say, "My God, I need you. My son is choking my wife." While those situations are scary, it's a double-sided coin because we are obligated to teach people to instead say, "My son is experiencing Tourette rage and threatening my wife." Putting handcuffs onto someone experiencing Tourette rage is going to exacerbate that situation and make it 100 times worse. Therefore, the best response is medical intervention rather than calling in law enforcement. I am trying to train the folks in South Carolina to revise how they handle these situations, so it doesn't end up in an arrest. Hopefully, that will happen when enough law enforcement officers learn about Tourette rage and really understand it.

To make a comparison to another condition, there is rage that goes along with autism as well. However, in my opinion, there's so much more protection around people who have this condition. The Autism Society, for instance, pays people to do advocacy work for them versus the Tourette Association, who expects people to do it on their own dime. However, the flip side of this — which I appreciate — is that the advocacy work is then more authentic. Yet, while the occurrences are very much the same, which is around one in fifty, autism is much more of a household word. I went to high school with an attorney for the Autism Society. She went to every single state and lobbied for autism coverage insurance. While this was no small feat, she got her bill passed in every single state. Her effort to pass such an important initiative made all the difference in the world to protect people afflicted by autism.

Jason Michaels: Well, that's incredible and crazy that the public perceives autism as being more important than Tourette's, especially when there are so many great people who work very hard to get the word out about Tourette education. I think if you compared education levels about autism versus Tourette Syndrome, the difference would be dramatic. While I don't want to offend teachers, many are much more educated about the former as opposed to the latter. They wouldn't think twice if you said, "I have an autistic child and need you to treat or interact with them in this way."

This contrasts with Tourette's where, while shameful and offensive, a school might say, "Let's get rid of this student because they're a pain." I would love to see more action and education around Tourette's. While it is way better now than it used to be, it's still not as good as one would hope.

Heather Ramsey: More action definitely needs to be taken. I've been on this journey since 2009 when Jacob was diagnosed. Some of the situations that I've encountered have been really challenging, but then there have been amazing opportunities like meeting you, and us doing the Zoom program* we did during COVID. That was amazing.

Most of all, I love the connections and people I've met, many of whom are outside of my network. Some of my best friends are not locals, but rather people I've met through the Tourette Assoication who live all over the country. It's amazing to know that there's a network of people who "get it" and "understand it." I want that same support system for others so they can also experience the joy that I have because of Tourette Syndrome.

Jason Michaels: That's amazing.

Heather Ramsey: You wouldn't think those two things would be in the same sentence.

Jason Michaels: Tell me just a little bit more about that. As I have said, you may look at Tourette Syndrome as the worst thing that's ever happened to you. Yet, in the future, you might look back at it as a gift. I want to dive into joy, because that is the opposite of what most people would associate with Tourette Syndrome.

Heather Ramsey: I agree. When my son was diagnosed in 2009, we were given a thirty-four page report where the doctor advised on the final page, "I encourage you to reach out to the Tourette Association of America, which has lots of resources." For that, I'm very grateful. I went to their website and saw that there was a conference happening the following March. I immediately told my husband, "We need to go as a family. I'll take the responsibility of doing the training, and y'all can spend your time sightseeing and stuff." And he said, "Okay."

The conference was Thursday through Sunday beginning with a seminar for those who were newly diagnosed with the condition. It was led by Dr. John Walkup. Now, Dr. Walkup is my idol, my hero. An amazing man, he is the expert in Tourette Syndrome and considered a guru in the field. That day convinced me of all of that. I did an eight-hour intensive deep dive into what Tourette's is and how it affects everything from medical to everyday situations. It was mind-boggling how incredible that information was. As I left, I said, "I want this same level of understanding for everybody." From there, I did more training, which taught me how to explain the condition to school staff and ask for the help that I needed. Most importantly, I met other people with Tourette Syndrome and families who could relate to the emotions and experiences I had lived. And I was like, "Wow, okay, that's cool."

The conference is biennial, which means it skipped a year. All I know is that I kept saying to my family, "I've got to go back." Fortunately, we made this happen — and while they indulged in vacation activities — I attended the trainings. There I met some truly incredible people including Dave Pittman*.

Jason Michaels: I know Dave!

Heather Ramsey: He came to North Carolina. As you know, his platform is anti-bullying, and he spoke to six different schools in our area during Anti-Bullying Awareness Month. It was amazing to bring him here for educational seminars and to sing for everybody.

Jason Michaels: Were there any programs your children participated in that gave them more strength and self-esteem?

Heather Ramsey: In 2013, I learned about the Tourette Association's youth ambassador program. My son said, "I want to do that," which led to a long-term involvement. Through that program, we met some amazing people and started solidifying relationships with other families afflicted by Tourette's. Finally, my son started to realize that he wasn't alone and started feeling really connected to both himself and others. We've continued to attend every March, whether there is a conference happening or not. The last day, and perhaps the most impactful, is when we advocate for Tourette's on Capitol Hill. There, we encourage the CDC to acquire more support and funding for Tourette Syndrome.

In 2016, my daughter Jordan finally joined our cause after expressing that she also wanted to become a youth ambassador. The three of us trained every year together until COVID hit. That's when the Tourette Association asked us to take our knowledge and step into the role of training other youth ambassadors. Besides the thrill of being a part of the association for so long, it was so special to see our experience come full circle. To transition, alongside my children, from a conference attendee to a teacher is the real success story.

Jason Michaels: And best of all, you're making a direct impact on people's lives.

Heather Ramsey: Exactly. Our experience is proof that when you do for others, you get back so much more than you give.

Jason Michaels: You are an incredible example of someone who is fighting the fight so hard. A few minutes ago, we spoke about how there needs to be more education, but you are literally doing it. You are actively putting in the time to create more education. The fact that I can ask a school group, "Who's heard of Tourette Syndrome?" and almost every single person raises their hand is thanks to you, your family, and countless others who are fighting the fight.

The Tourette community owes you a big thank you, not just for your work, but your passion as well. And that's a big deal. If you were getting paid for your efforts, it would still be impressive. But the fact that you are willingly giving your time for the greater good deserves a round of applause. There are people you may never meet whom you have impacted.

Heather Ramsey: I hope so.

Jason Michaels: Oh, there's no question. Think about it from this angle: While the direct impact of your work may not always be tangible, a teacher that you educate today could use your techniques ten years down the line.

Heather Ramsey: Yeah, that's true. That made me think of one more success story that I would like to share.

Jason Michaels: Give it to me.

Heather Ramsey: Well, I have two. As you know, I love full circle situations such as the fact that you did a Zoom program for us on June 4, which is Tourette Awareness Day in North and South Carolina. I've been requesting proclamations for this observance since 2015. Previous to this, no one had tried to officially commemorate it. We're now up to sixty-four towns in North and South Carolina that proclaim this as a day of awareness every year. This achievement is something I'm very excited and passionate about.

In the town that I live in, the mayor has always been supportive. Every year he presents the proclamation at the meeting. He even lets me say a few words about the intention behind it. We have an official photo op and everything.

A couple of years ago, a local family had a member diagnosed with Tourette's. After hearing the mayor speak at an event and reading in his bio that one of his initiatives is Tourette Syndrome awareness, the dad decided to email him. He explained that his daughter had just been diagnosed with Tourette's, and he wanted to know more about how his office could support them. In the mayor's response, he copied me and said, "Heather is your person and can provide any information that you want." His daughter then became a youth ambassador who now goes with me to accept proclamations. Who would've thought that a local mayor would be integral to a family getting help for their daughter?

Jason Michaels: That's correct.

Heather Ramsey: Another full circle success story that I would love to share involves encouraging someone close to me to change her career path. During COVID, my mother lived with us for eighteen months due to her health, which led to us employing home health services. Of all the specialists, the occupational therapist and I just clicked on a personal level. We were usually her last appointment of the day, and she would usually stay for cocktails afterwards. As she came in and out over many weeks, she became aware of my advocacy work. I eventually told her about Comprehensive Behavioral Intervention for Tics (CBIT) as it's the only non-pharmacological treatment for Tourette Syndrome. "You should look into this as an occupational therapist," I explained to her one day, "because there aren't very many who offer this in the United States. Also, since so few occupational therapists are trained in CBIT, insurance doesn't cover it, which makes it easier to take on new patients." Six months later, she emailed to confirm that she had done her training and needed an initial patient. "Will you be mine?" she asked.

Jason Michaels: Oh, wow.

Heather Ramsey: Okay, wow is right. My immediate thought was, ***While this is cool, I am not your person.*** At 53 years old I wasn't the right candidate because I had no interest in homework. However, I told her, "Because I love you, I will do it." Working with her on my breathing tic was the best thing I ever did. Now unless I get really stressed out, the breathing tic that has bothered me forever is pretty much gone. It also gives me such satisfaction to employ the competing response, which overpowers the tic. It's so exhilarating because I've tried lots of things and finally found one that works.

Jason Michaels: That's fantastic!

Heather Ramsey: I love how everything comes full circle.

Jason Michaels: It does. It's crazy how that works. Beautiful.

Heather Ramsey: Above all else, relationships with other Tourette families bring me the most joy. I so badly want that level of belonging and comfort for others. There is great strength that comes from connecting with others who've had the same experiences. You may think you're the only parent whose child has Tourette rage and punches you, is defiant, or lashes out. Then you realize ***Holy crap, there are hundreds of people in this same situation. I'm not a freak simply because it's impossible for most people to understand.*** My sisters and parents, who at one point in time were judgmental, have been particularly mind blown by the information I've shared with them. They used to say, "Oh, I'd never allow those kinds of outbursts," to which I would tell them, "That's like telling a paraplegic to walk. You don't get it." That's how it is, which is why support groups are so important. I encourage others to find that joy.

Jason Michaels: Just on a personal note, I can't wait for people to read this because I think it's going to impact them immensely.

Heather Ramsey: I agree 100%.

JASON'S SUMMARY

Heather is a wonderful example of someone putting other people's needs in front of her own. Her efforts advocating for others are heroic, and she deserves that distinction from the Tourette Syndrome community.

I was particularly struck by her comment early in the interview about being willing to talk openly and honestly about the condition. As a reminder, here is what she said:

"My husband is a very reserved and private person, who tips farther on the introverted scale than me. He said, 'I don't think we need to tell anybody.' When I started thinking about it, I thought: ***what message is that sending? If we are telling our son to fake it or suppress it, what kind of message is that sending?***"

I couldn't agree more with her decision to be transparent about his condition. Talking about it can be very difficult or feel embarrassing. Yet, to Heather's point, staying silent would set a tone of shame. Sometimes it is the hard things that we must do to overcome the challenges that we face.

"Talking about it," in the sense of being transparent about personal struggles, is so important that I highlight it as one of five major points in my keynote program on building Resiliency. Personally, when I started talking with others about me having Tourette's, I went from a place of feeling a great deal of embarrassment because of my tics — to a place where I realized that having Tourette's was perfectly normal for me, and that I was okay with it.

At one point in the interview, Heather also stated regarding her initial illiteracy about Tourette's, "On one hand, I feel incredibly guilty for not being better equipped to deal with my son. I was doing the best I could at the time, and I'm just grateful he's resilient."

I want to be very clear that I fully understand what Heather is saying. With that said, I believe that the best thing we can do is to learn from our prior ignorance so that we can educate more thoroughly and help others be more empathetic, exactly as Heather has done.

Guilt around a lack of awareness doesn't really serve anyone. What is more constructive is taking something you know very little about and becoming a subject matter expert in it. By helping thousands, Heather has set the standard for what we should all aim to achieve in life. As she said so eloquently, "I can help people now the way I wish I could have then."

Of particular note is Heather's work with people in positions of authority to help those of us with Tourette's be better understood by them. By being willing to talk about it, she is educating those of us with Tourette's how to deal with the police and the police how to best deal with emotional outbursts.

If you've ever wondered how you can help yourself, your loved one, or your friend with Tourette Syndrome, follow Heather's example and speak up, educate, and advocate. Subscribing to those three pillars is the best way that you can change the world for them.

Personally, I am outraged at the difference in visibility and education for those people living with autism versus those of us with Tourette's. If the numbers are the same, it's shameful that the Tourette's community hasn't done a better job mobilizing an aggressive team to work on our behalf. While I certainly don't want to minimize autism, the simple fact is that the Tourette community needs a much greater megaphone. We deserve far more advocates who can teach others about our identity, what we live with, and how we can become productive members of society. Only then will we reduce how often people living with Tourette's are laughed at or bullied by misinformed, small-minded people.

If you read the Nikki Burdine interview, you may recall that she also mentioned behavioral therapy. Consider this your giant flashing billboard to learn more about this excellent way to help with tics.

The final thing that stood out to me was when Heather spoke about the joy that she found forming relationships with other families of people with Tourette's. As humans, we were built to function at our best when in community. If you are in the States, one excellent place to look for community is the Tourette Association of America. There are similar organizations in other countries such as Tourette's Action in the United Kingdom and the Tourette Syndrome Association of Australia.

If you are looking to connect with a community of like-minded individuals living with Tourette Syndrome, and their families and friends, you are also welcome to join my online Tourette Warrior community.

For more information, please visit www.TouretteWarrior.com

---

*A 504 student is a child with a physical or mental impairment that substantially limits one or more major life activities (e.g., learning, concentrating, breathing), entitled to legally binding accommodations under Section 504 of the Rehabilitation Act. These plans ensure equal access to education without requiring specialized instruction.

*Coprolalia is the involuntary, uncontrollable, and repetitive utterance of obscene, taboo, or socially inappropriate words and phrases.

*In 2020, I partnered with Tourette groups to present a virtual program where I performed magic and shared my story of growing up with Tourette's to support the Tourette's community.

*Dave Pittman is a Christian musician who lives with Tourette Syndrome. His story is told later in this book.

To watch the video of the full interview with Heather Ramsey, access additional tools to help you live and thrive with Tourette Syndrome, and connect with the Tourette Warrior community, please visit TouretteWarrior.com.

In the next chapter, I interview Jack Cordwell who shares how a strong work ethic made him an invaluable, in-demand member of a team. He also discusses the technique that he used to "time travel," and in a very heartfelt moment, shares his most important parenting messages with his son.

CHAPTER 3

JACK CORDWELL

ATTORNEY

Jack Cordwell is an attorney who lives with Tourette Syndrome. He is a powerful example of how living resiliently can set us up for success in life. There are some wonderful lessons that Jack had to learn "the hard way" that he graciously shares with us.

Jason Michaels: I'd like you to tell the story of how we met because I love how we first connected.

Jack Cordwell: My buddy and I are regulars at Zanies comedy club in Nashville, Tennessee. We have this habit of always sitting on the bottom floor. For whatever reason, we happened to be up top in the balcony one evening, which was an interesting experience on its own. As I was walking out, I saw you ticcing which stopped me in my tracks because I don't run across too many people with Tourette Syndrome. I thought, I've got to go talk to that guy. My buddy kept on walking while I debated on whether I should talk to you. Finally, after chickening out a few times, I turned back around and literally interrupted your conversation. The funny thing is that was the first time I ever did anything like that.

Jason Michaels: I remember it well, because when you asked about my Tourette's, it surprised me.

Jack Cordwell: There was an instant familiarity. I've had people confront me my entire life about my tics; however, I've never had the opportunity to say to somebody, "Hey, I recognize your condition because I have this too." That was weird in a good way. While approaching you was an entirely different way of behaving for me, it was easier than I thought — a new experience.

Jason Michaels: And you know what? I remember after I was diagnosed as a kid and looking around my school wondering if there were other people like me. There might've been some folks … maybe, but I didn't see anybody that I could tell who was having tics.

I remember going to my church with my family one time and saying, “Hey, let's sit down front.” My Mom responded, “Would you rather sit in the back?” And I was like, “We can sit wherever.” It wasn't until later, when we were talking, that she admitted, “I didn't want you to be in a situation where people would be staring at you and potentially making you feel uncomfortable.” It made me think, “Oh, is that why we sat in the back for so long?” (Laughs.) Because I didn't know. We weren't back row Baptists. We were trying to keep me out of a situation in which people might stare at me, or point, or whisper, or laugh at me. I was fortunate to have protective parents who were looking out for me.

Jack Cordwell: My experience is very different as I wasn't diagnosed until I was 21. The person who encouraged me to go see a specialist had already done the research. We already knew what the diagnosis was. The appointment was really just to confirm it and then see if there was anything I could do.

When I was growing up, there was always a question of, “What's wrong with you?” surrounding my behavior. I'd seen people with tics and nervous habits, but not Tourette's.

As a kid in rural Florida, I grew up playing sports, like many of my elementary school peers, and performing in plays. My love for singing started in church. In high school, I was fortunate to be able to sing in a variety of venues; however, I was always placed in the back. At the time, I assumed this was because I was a terrible dancer. Yet, in my senior year of high school I finally saw myself on video doing a full facial squint from the back row. I was like, “Oh that's what my tics look like.”

Jason Michaels: Wow. That's an eye-opening moment, no pun intended.

Jack Cordwell: Yeah, I've thought a lot about that. I was very active in theater to the point that I was on a scholarship for a show choir my first two years of college. We toured and did thirty-five shows a year, which was a lot of fun. We even performed on a cruise the two summers that I was with them. For one reason or another, I gave up on acting and instead decided to build sets so I could stay in the theater world. Set building really called to me so I immersed myself in that. Then I transferred to a college in West Tennessee where I got involved in their theater program. I was in a show and one day the director turned to me and rudely asked, "Why do you keep doing that thing with your face?"

I said, "What do you mean?" to which he responded, "The eyes thing. Can you stop that?" I confirmed that I had always done that tic; however, I would try to stop. It was particularly frustrating because he kept insisting that he had never seen it before. The bottom line was, he wanted me to stop. And I could stop the tics when I focused really hard and was immersed in my character. Then, they weren't as prevalent. However, when I was in the back or not focused, the tics would happen. These included a plethora of tics from a head shake to a full facial squint that I am still uncomfortable talking about at times.

Jason Michaels: Yeah, absolutely. The most interesting element of your story is that it aligns with my theory: The Tourette's community is very creative and filled with tons of artists, singers, and performers. For whatever reason, that seems to be the pattern that keeps showing up.

Jack Cordwell: I wonder if it has to do with the fact that we study people? We know that we're different and are therefore trying to see what is normal. If what I'm doing is atypical, then what is everyone else like?

I spend a lot of time trying to mask my tics particularly as an attorney. When I was in front of an audience, in court for example, I had to be even more aware of my tics and their focus. I couldn't let anyone think that because I was nodding my head, I was agreeable to what they had said. That head shake tic would look like I was in accordance with their belief. So, I would try to be animated in hopes that moving around a lot would disguise it.

Jason Michaels: Even as a fully grown, mature adult, I still mask my tics out of self-protection. I might be walking down the grocery store aisle on a Saturday afternoon, and some stranger will ask, "Are you okay?" Instead of trying to educate them on my tics I just say, "Yep, I'm fine" while I rub my neck and pretend that I pulled a muscle in it. It gets exhausting having to brief people on your condition every single time.

Jack Cordwell: Yes, it can be an exhausting proposition to bring new people into your world. In business, I'm "on." You're "on." We're focused. While that focus is greatly beneficial when you are meeting new people, you can't be in that state all day long. It's too tiring.

Jason Michaels: Right.

Jack Cordwell: A lot of people, when I finally tell them that I have Tourette's, say, "Well, I didn't notice anything." I am not sure how this could be true since I am the kind of person who closely watches other people's mannerisms. Maybe they're being kind, or maybe they really didn't notice. I don't know.

Jason Michaels: I remember one time years ago, while in a busy grocery store, being very aware that I was looking around to see if anybody was noticing my tics. At that specific moment, it did not appear as though anybody was paying any attention to me. They were all very focused on finding the next item on their grocery lists. This sparked a realization that people are so in their own worlds, they're not paying that much attention to what's happening around them.

Jack Cordwell: I have noticed something similar, which is people seem to select what they focus on or ignore. This became especially noticeable to me because I come from two dramatically different worlds: construction, which I grew up in, and the business world I work in now.

When I was in construction, we didn't have a uniform. You wore old clothes because you weren't going to wear your fancy suit to dig a ditch, move concrete, or clean up a job site. You looked rough.

Still, as an adult, it's fairly normal for me to put on a pair of stained jeans and a shirt with some holes in it. Sometimes I've gone out covered in grease, like this one time, when I went into the grocery store after riding around in my bulldozer. Honestly, I didn't realize how bad I looked until I realized that people wouldn't make eye contact with me because of my appearance.

Jason Michaels: It's interesting how appearance can change people's behavior.

Jack Cordwell: They were very uncomfortable. On the opposite end of the spectrum, after attending an event I walked into Home Depot one day. I was looking fancy in my sports coat, slacks, and freshly pressed button-down shirt. While I cannot remember what aisle I was in, I do recall that I had two five-gallon buckets of drywall compound, one in each hand. As I was walking towards the cashier, this guy jumps over the counter and says, "Sir, let me help you."

Completely excluding Tourette's, I find it interesting what people notice, particularly as it's related to appearance or behavior. Certain cues that one person picks up on, another might ignore entirely. I can almost see the wheels turning in people's heads as they notice something in their peripheral vision and go, ***Yeah, I don't really want to pay attention to that.***

Jason Michaels: Since you were diagnosed as an adult, did you find yourself masking right away? Or rather, did it always feel normal to find natural movements that deflected attention away from your tics? I would imagine, especially if people like that teacher criticized you, masking became a form of self-protection. Does that sound accurate?

Jack Cordwell: Probably. I remember as a nine or ten year old who played football, I had to wear a mouthpiece with a plastic guard. It entirely hid my mouth like a dirt shield. I must have done a lip curl or something similar because, suddenly, the coach smacked me on the helmet and said, "Don't smile when I'm talking to you!" Even though I tried to defend myself and explain that I wasn't smiling, but was rather doing a tic, he didn't want to hear it. He was freaked out and basically said, "Go away."

Jason Michaels: Yeah, that sounds like how things were back in the 1980's and 90's.

Jack Cordwell: I also had a family member who was determined to break me free from my nervous habits. That was a tough situation where I think they meant well. I honestly believe they thought they were doing something beneficial by saying, "I'll take care of this. I'm going to handle this." Every day they would follow me around and just constantly say, "Stop doing that" repeatedly. Even worse, I had three tics then that included blinking really fast, snapping, and lip curling.

I used to have the same conversation with people all the time who felt they had a solution for me. I had one person ask me if I got hit in the head and maybe that was the reason for my tics because they knew somebody one time who got hit in the head as an adult. They wondered if that was maybe what was wrong with me. Or maybe I had a vitamin A deficiency? "Did I wear contacts?" was a regular one with the blinking tic. They would say, "Are your eyes dry?" to which I would respond, "No, I don't wear contacts." Immediately after asking, they would justify their question by saying, "Well, I'm just trying to help." That was probably the common denominator, right? A lot of people really mean well. I sincerely believe their inquiries were intended to help me be normal for my benefit.

Maybe if I could be more like them, I would have an easier life. Yet the truth is that people know very little about Tourette's. Even though they comment on it, they don't understand it. Oftentimes, it feels like their education comes from a joke that a comedian made at some point in time. That's how I sincerely believe most people pick up on it.

Jason Michaels: Was there ever a time when someone unexpectedly inserted themselves, and it actually improved the situation?

Jack Cordwell: A friend, who had never known anyone with Tourette's prior to me, was working out at the gym one day. One of the other gym members who was there had a t-shirt on that showed someone exhibiting profane behavior. Basically, in a very derogatory way, it was making fun of coprolalia. "Let's just pretend I have Tourette's" was written across the front of the t-shirt justifying the behavior. This apparently upset my friend so much that she went up to him and said, "That's not nice." While I would never ask or suggest what someone else should do, it was comforting to know I had another advocate in my corner. In a way, it confirmed that she understood how incredibly difficult my path is. Unfortunately, there is no medication that will make it all go away.

Jason Michaels: There's a lot right there to unpack. First off, having a family member break you of a "bad habit" to "help" you could ultimately affect somebody's long term mental health.

Then you've got people who are genuinely trying to help figure out the source of your tics. While they might have the best intentions, I can only imagine how embarrassing that would be. Personally, I would never want other people constantly pointing out my tics or talking about them. If I'm being honest, it sounds like you had to deal with a lot of crap which I don't want to sugarcoat for the sake of others.

Jack Cordwell: Yeah, it wasn't fun.

Jason Michaels: There will be people who will read this and feel less alone because they'll think, ***Wait a minute. I'm not the only person who had to deal with this.*** You've also been bullied by teachers, an experience other people with Tourette's might relate to. Unfortunately, there are too many professionals who are unaware, uneducated, or ignorant. Some teachers, like the ones you dealt with, might even choose not to acknowledge your condition because they don't believe that tics are possible. Yet, despite all of this, you've become an adult who can deal with different people in different settings. You've made life work for yourself: from your business, to your friends, to the theater life that I know you still love. A child or young person with Tourette's might look at their situation and think, "There is no tomorrow, because how is my life ever going to change?" Yet you, Jack, are a perfect example of somebody who has dealt with some very difficult situations and come out of them admirably. You have advanced degrees, and you are a very intelligent and successful person. You are thriving as an adult. The world, especially children, needs examples of people like that.

Jack Cordwell: Those are very kind words that you're offering, but I've never looked at it that way. I've had conversations with my own children about how being the kid who must work a little harder than everyone else isn't a bad thing because it gives you grit. The thing that I learned very young was how to enjoy working. It didn't matter what the task was, because many of them were not that enjoyable. They simply had to be done. And I'm not referring to schoolwork kind of tasks. Because I worked whenever school was out. A good example is when I was on the job site with my father. I worked. When I was younger, maybe I didn't accomplish all that much, but there was always work that I could focus on. Then as I got older, there were always big tasks to be completed. So, I would set these challenges for myself and make games out of the work. I think that Tourette's was always a part of it, right? I don't know what it's like without that.

Jason Michaels: How did the challenges you faced shape your personality.

Jack Cordwell: My hobbies, they tend to be solitary ones. I have a woodworking shop, and I taught myself how to weld during the pandemic. You don't normally have a lot of people around unless you're paying somebody to help you. Yet, I really enjoy woodworking in particular and watching things come together. Lately, as you mentioned, I was given a wonderful opportunity to revisit the theater and assist my daughter's school as a set builder. My personality might be a little more driven and perfectionistic than most. There's always that thought running through my mind saying gotta get it right, gotta get it right. However, I am working through that quirk and accepting the fact that it comes along with my intense focus. If there was a bright line that came out of Tourette's, it was the ability to hyper focus. That focus is what it took to get around the tics to complete anything — especially in high school.

Jason Michaels: Let's say you were talking to a younger version of yourself; do you have any advice or a point of view that you would share with that person?

Jack Cordwell: Let me tell you a story. I was having a conversation with my son. He was sitting in that chair right there a couple of years ago. I said, "If I could go back and talk to myself," which was a lengthy conversation that led to the meaning of parenting crystallizing. I continued, "I'm a time traveler because even though we are in the same room, I am you from the future." Then I talked to him about the things that matter. I said, "This is the closest that anyone can get to time travel, telling their child, 'Danger, danger, Will Robinson.' Maybe the reference was lost on him*, but I felt like I could teach him the things to focus on. Don't get carried away with this right here because it will happen eventually. Have fun and enjoy yourself. However, always remember that the point of school is to set yourself up for the future." To circle back to your original question, I've already thought about the advice I would give because I said it to my son.

Jason Michaels: That's great.

Jack Cordwell: Unfortunately, my younger self doesn't get to benefit, but my current self does because I watch my son and my daughter develop by listening to my lessons. Both have been fortunate not to have Tourette's that I can tell.

Long ago I accepted that this is it. There's only so much I can control with Tourette's. What am I going to do now? How am I going to move forward? In some ways, I had to be better than other people to get opportunities even if it was just singing in the back. Sometimes the opportunity was that, yes, I got to sing, but I got placed in the back. If there was a task to be done in my desired arena, I would not only take it on but also become exceptionally good at it. My goal was to make myself invaluable. Then I would be needed, and nobody would focus on my tics.

Jason Michaels: Were there any masking behaviors you used that helped draw attention away from the tics?

Jack Cordwell: Probably my biggest masking tic, as ironic as it sounds, was looking someone directly in the eye when talking to them. If I could capture their attention, eventually they would look away and I could tic. People can only engage for so long. While my eye contact was probably unusually intense, that's one way I covered up my tics.

While it's hard at this stage in life to openly tic, I'm sure I do anyway. I spent the early part of my legal career in court arguing in front of judges and trying to capture their attention without being distracting. Unfortunately, I dressed the part, fastening my tie really tight around my collar. This essentially choked my neck, which triggered tics badly. I would leave court in massive pain from just trying to hold tight and stand still. Fortunately, I didn't have to worry about a jury staring at me because it was rare that I worked with them. Yet, when I was the center of attention, I had to make sure that my responses weren't perceived as being in agreement with someone. That is probably when my theater training kicked in, and I decided to be very animated in order to mask my head tic.

Jason Michaels: That's a very high stress situation.

Jack Cordwell: In my first position, the attorney that hired me said, "I picked you because your resume stated that you were a theater major in college." As he had never hired another attorney with a theater background, he wanted to see what it would be like. My first reaction was "Yay! That degree finally paid off."

Jason Michaels: Getting back to wisdom gleaned from experience, if you were talking to parents of a child with Tourette Syndrome, what do you want them to know?

Jack Cordwell: Treat them like they're normal. Don't sit in the back of the church. Well-meaning can be dangerous because what does it mean anyways? I would tell parents to stick to a plan, which means honesty. Don't sugarcoat the condition and say, "Everything's going to be great." Don't hide your child. The best way for them to become more accepting of it is to live their life. You don't get better at sports by watching a bunch of videos. You get better at sports by playing them.

Jason Michaels: Yep.

Jack Cordwell: You can only educate yourself so much until you finally have to get out there and do it. Your parents' approach obviously worked based on the fact that you're a performer who isn't afraid to be in front of people. You don't hide, so obviously the path they took was a successful one for you.

Jason Michaels: Well, you know what? They took your advice before you gave it in the sense that they pretty much treated me like normal. While they may have eliminated certain situations that would've led to me being ostracized or alienated, I pretty much had a typical childhood. So, I think your advice is spot on and echoes what I would also want to say.

To lighten up the mood a bit, do you have any funny stories about Tourette Syndrome? While that might sound weird, it's such a serious topic that I would love to hear about a time when you looked back and thought, "That's kind of funny."

Jack Cordwell: In college, I was in the commons one day sitting down talking and playing cards. In all honesty, I was probably trying to meet girls. All of a sudden, a girl walked by me and winked. It was a huge wink — with both eyes possibly. Immediately, I thought, ***Who is that?!*** That was the girl I ended up marrying.

Jason Michaels: Oh! (Laughing.)

Jack Cordwell: I asked her about that before our wedding day and she said, "Well, I thought you were winking at me, so I winked back."

Jason Michaels: Oh my gosh, that's crazy.

Jack Cordwell: Go tic!

I have echolalia*, which oftentimes gives people very random tics. For example, I would mimic my wife's accent, which was very Southern at the time. For years she said, "I thought you were just teasing me," when in actuality that was a tic. In a way, not understanding the reason behind my behavior probably made it easier to accept. Back then, there was no book. We had nothing. All I wanted were answers to simple questions like, "What is the range of tics with this particular condition?" or, "Why can't I focus?" and finally, "Why can't I stop?"

Jason Michaels: Yes, I also know what it is like to shake your head and wonder why do I behave this way?

Jack Cordwell: Still, here's one more funny story. Back in the early 2000's, I was hired as a carpenter. One of my clients flew me down South to work on a house he'd purchased for his daughter in Orlando, Florida. Towards the end of the project, it was clear that I lacked time for the painting part. He said, "Can you hire one to complete the job?" to which I said, "Sure." From there, I called one of my buddies, an accomplished painter, to paint while I finished building cabinets. He followed right behind me.

On our final day, as we cleaned up the tools, I noticed that a few five-gallon buckets had lines of paint on the side. I said, “Alright, let’s clean these down” to which he said, “Just let them dry. They’ll be fine.” However, I kept insisting that I had to do this even after he explained that we might miss the plane. “No man, I’ve got to clean these buckets” is what I kept saying. I knew it wouldn’t take me long and I had to complete that task. What I have realized since then is that obsessive compulsiveness tends to kick in when I am overtired. When I am exhausted, that need kicks in. “Fine, we’ll clean the buckets,” he finally said. We’ve had a conversation about the situation since, which he summarized as, “I think I understand now that you weren’t going to stop.” What I’ve learned about myself is that sometimes, even though I don’t want to, I have to tic. I don’t want to, but I just can’t stop it. Managing the tic is one thing, but trying to stop it completely is too much. That OCD episode was not a tic, but it is a thing. Yet, that’s a whole other story, right?

Jason Michaels: Can you explain that further?

Jack Cordwell: I've noticed that sometimes I just have to allow myself to release that energy. I don't think anything bad’s going to happen to anybody if I don’t. It’s just that I intuitively know that something else will pop up. That’s a lot of managing. It’s easier to just make eye contact with somebody and let the tics happen when nobody’s looking.

Jason Michaels: If you had to think of a single superpower you’ve developed thanks to Tourette Syndrome, what would you say it is?

Jack Cordwell: Awareness. I had a friend who pointed out this hypersensitivity a few years ago. I have a more profound ability than most to pay attention to everything around me. This includes studying people and watching subtle changes in their mood. All of it comes back to self-protection. If I know how others act, then I’ll understand how much to let out. There is an extreme sense of awareness when it comes to what is happening all around me.

Jason Michaels: I would say that's definitely a superpower.

Jack Cordwell: The flip side of the coin is that hurtful things can stay in your mind forever. When I was in high school, teachers told me they'd be happy if I graduated high school. At the end of my freshman year my counselor said, "What classes do you want to take?" I told him I was ready to move on to geometry because it was a university prerequisite. Instead of being impressed he said, "You're not college material and might instead want to think about trade school. That's probably a better path for you." When I questioned his opinion all he said was, "I'm looking at your grades, and it would just be more realistic." What do you say to that? I thought ***Oh, okay.***

Jason Michaels: Wow.

Jack Cordwell: His lack of faith in my abilities affected me, for sure. I mean, I still took the classes I had intended to take. I still struggled through them and had to work really hard just to get by. It wasn't until I went to law school that it all kind of made sense. I honestly felt like I was a decade behind, which I guess I was, because I started at age thirty-two. None of it made sense in high school. College sort of didn't make sense, and that's another story in and of itself. Yet, law school was different, not due to how intensely I focused, but rather how badly I wanted it.

Law school, in many ways, was its own thing. That experience had its own unique path. You started here, and if you worked hard enough, maybe you could get to here. I looked for others with that same drive. As much as graduate studies mostly fall on your own shoulders, I found myself communing with others. We got far simply by inspiring one another. Other days, I needed friends who could push me and say, "Dude, you're messing up!" I had a very good friend in law school who often gave me that very message, yet using more colorful words.

While beyond challenging, the logic of law school at least made sense to me. I enjoyed the practicality of it and the conversations that came along with my classmates. Really, I enjoyed every part. The difficult parts were approached with acceptance. "Of course it's difficult, but this is something you've got to do." As I tried to remind myself daily, if nothing had been easy so far, why would this be? Why would I keep going if it was? So, instead I chose to enjoy the entire process of studying law. While there were aspects, such as teachers that made it tough, earning that degree was worth it.

Jason Michaels: The best part of all is that it was your own path. Law school was what made sense to you at the time. And I guarantee somebody reading this, thanks to your sincerity, will say, "You know what? That is my path too. His words speak to me."

Jack Cordwell: Do you remember the 1980s TV show "L.A. Law?"

Jason Michaels: Oh, yeah, I remember that show.

Jack Cordwell: I remember this particular episode where this lawyer would walk around spouting awful words. They fired him because of this bad behavior, which turned out to be Tourette Syndrome. Ultimately, they came to a compromise because he said, "Look I can't control this, but I do not want to be fired. I love the law." The compromise they came up with was that he would work from home, even before that was a thing.

Yet, what is upsetting about this memory is that coprolalia isn't the only explanation of Tourette Syndrome. While that was probably forty years ago, I still think it would've been nice to have been nine years old and had a better role model for what I was dealing with. Maybe I would be different from who I am today. That extra consideration might have helped soften some rough edges.

Ultimately, there was no one to look up to, and I had to be the one to navigate it. As a kid, teenager, and adult I had to learn how to handle and control my own behavior. The truth is, I like people and having conversations too much to ever be satisfied working from home.

Jason Michaels: Oh, man, this is great. Let me just say "thank you" again. After doing a number of these interviews, I've realized there are certain moments where I get hit by the feeling ***Wow, somebody needs to hear this message right now!*** It happened multiple times while we've been speaking, and I am just very appreciative of your willingness, time, and vulnerability. The open way in which you approached this interview isn't always easy so much gratitude to you.

Jack Cordwell: Well, I haven't sought out opportunities to commune with other people in the Tourette community. Yet, especially after having this conversation, I believe more than ever that we need to seek each other out. It is essential to support one another. It is easy to get carried away in your own life because our existence can be very hard. However, I am the one who's appreciative, both for the opportunity to be featured, but also because you're doing exactly what is needed.

JASON’S SUMMARY

There are numerous lessons that I take away from the interview with Jack. With that said, one main idea seemed to be a recurring theme, which revolved around hard work.

Early in the interview Jack said, “I've had conversations with my own children about how being the kid who must work a little harder than everyone else isn’t a bad thing because it gives you grit. The thing that I learned very young was how to enjoy working. It didn't matter what the task was, because many of them were not that enjoyable.”

This may not be the lesson that everyone wants to hear, but I think it’s important to understand that sometimes, to get ahead in life, we have to be focused on simply “doing the work.”

In fact, setting a goal and then doing the hard, sometimes unenjoyable work, is how you become accomplished. Goals are often achieved by doing the work others don’t want to do.

Want to get ahead in life? Do the work. Equating “work” with being a means to an end is an advanced form of resilient thinking.

Jack followed up on those comments later in the interview when he said, “If there was a task to be done in my desired arena, I would not only take it on but also become exceptionally good at it. My goal was to make myself invaluable. Then I would be needed, and nobody would focus on my tics.”

This is another excellent strategy for how to be successful in life. Learning a skill that others don’t have and becoming really good at it makes you an extremely valuable member of a team. When both of those things occur, your confidence grows, too.

One of the reasons that I chose to write this book is because I didn’t want someone with Tourette Syndrome to listen to the doubters. Why should anyone with a dream allow the naysayers to discourage them?

That is why Jack's story of being told as a high school student that he would never go to college is such a powerful example of resilience and self-belief.

My mind is blown — and not in a good way — when I hear stories of people like Jack being told they will never accomplish a goal that they are considering. I'm so glad that Jack Cordwell stands as a powerful example of what can happen when doubters are ignored. Just like Jack, we simply "do the work" to become the person we aspire to be.

On another note, I found Jack's advice on accepting your tics to be revolutionary. As he said, "Don't hide your child. The best way for them to become more accepting of it is to live their life. You don't get better at sports by watching a bunch of videos. You get better at sports by playing them."

It's not always easy to have that mindset. When tics are overwhelming and the world is cruel, it can be very difficult to have that point of view. That advice, though, does track with who Jack is. He is a man who believes in living authentically even if it risks making himself or others slightly uncomfortable at times. To try to fight his tics would be like Jack pretending to be someone else.

Jack's advice reminds me of a famous quote from Theodore Roosevelt, "It is not the critic who counts: not the man who points out how the strong man stumbles or where the doer of deeds could have done better. The credit belongs to the man who is actually in the arena, whose face is marred by dust and sweat and blood, who strives valiantly, who errs and comes up short again and again, because there is no effort without error or shortcoming, but who knows the great enthusiasms, the great devotions, who spends himself in a worthy cause; who, at the best, knows, in the end, the triumph of high achievement, and who, at the worst, if he fails, at least he fails while daring greatly, so that his place shall never be with those cold and timid souls who knew neither victory nor defeat.*"

Every one of us who has ever struggled to live the life that we want to live, and not the life that someone else wanted us to live, should remember this quote and refer to it frequently.

Finally, I love what Jack said about seeking support when you have a somewhat isolating condition. As someone who did not seek "opportunities to commune with other people in the Tourette community. Yet, especially after having this conversation, I believe more than ever that we need to seek each other out. It is essential to support one another."

Connecting with others who have similar life experiences helps us gain perspective. It also gives us a network of people we can talk to and learn from. By living in community, we can shorten our own learning curve and help "normalize" living with tics. Shared knowledge is what this book is about after all.

---

* "Danger, danger, Will Robinson" is a popular expression from the 1960s television show "Lost In Space."

*Echolalia is the unsolicited, automatic repetition of words, phrases, or sounds heard from others (immediate) or recalled from memory (delayed).

*This quote came from Theodore Roosevelt's famous speech often called "Citizenship in a Republic." He delivered it on April 23, 1910, in Paris at the Sorbonne University during his post-presidency European tour. (Chat GPT)

To watch the video of the full interview with Jack Cordwell, access additional tools to help you live and thrive with Tourette Syndrome, and connect with the Tourette Warrior community, please visit TouretteWarrior.com.

In the next chapter, the interview with 911 Dispatcher Andrew Dalholt, Andrew talks about stress management and his outlook that the majority of the TS tics he dealt with were mostly just "annoying."

CHAPTER 4

ANDREW DALHOLT

911 DISPATCHER

Andrew Dalholt is a 911 Dispatcher, which is a high-stress job where he has to keep his cool under difficult circumstances. The nature of Andrew's work means that people in distress count on him to be calm, cool, and collected during their most intense moments of need. Andrew is a great example of someone with Tourette Syndrome who learned to manage his condition so he could be a source of help for people in difficult situations. In turn, he gave himself the freedom to follow his dream and succeed at the highest level possible.

Jason Michaels: Andrew, tell me about yourself and what you do.

Andrew Dalholt: I am a 911 dispatcher where the bulk of my duties is call taking. I pick up the phone calls from 911 lines, and I help people on the scene. I get the resources out and help them as fast as I can.

Then there's the fire station where I work as well. There I work on the radio for Fire EMS units. All day long, I'm talking with firefighters and medical response. The call taker puts in the call, which means we get all of the necessary information, like an address, before I assign the right units and get them out to that location. Then there's the police channel as well, which is the same idea, but for all the police units. I figure out what police units need to go where and talk with the police.

There's a system that I work on — which is an international system that is also a part of the FBI. It's all tied into one. So, when a judge issues a warrant, you enter the information into the system. That way if an officer comes to your channel and is like, "Hey, we're out with this person," I run their name through the system and check their history for guns or illegal activity.

We rotate through all those stations. It's just to keep everything fresh and new so we don't get stagnant on things the entire time we are at work.

Jason Michaels: It sounds like there are times when it could be very high stress.

Andrew Dalholt: Oh, for sure.

Jason Michaels: How do you stay calm as someone who is in the midst of chaos and trying to keep a relative stranger relaxed? On top of that, you're also trying to make sure all the information gets to the right place. As someone with Tourette Syndrome, does it affect your tics when you're in these types of live wire situations?

Andrew Dalholt: I still technically have Tourette's, but a lot of it has lessened from my childhood. As of now, I could count the ways in which Tourette's affects my daily life on one hand. Now my symptoms are very minor versus in my childhood when it was first diagnosed.

When I'm working the job, I do a lot of general stress management. I feel like I would be a lot more stressed if I was on the scene. At least I know I have access to resources to help someone in a majority of the situations we deal with without being directly involved in the action. Knowing that brings down my stress levels. I also send professionals to assess the scene in person. Overall, I am not as stressed as people would assume because I have a number of manuals with different medical procedures that can be done over the line, and different protocols to keep the party safe. I do whatever needs to be done in the moment I am privy to. So, I think I'm not as stressed on calls as people would assume because we have so many resources for every situation.

Jason Michaels: You made mention that there are certain stress management techniques that have also helped you. Are these things that were taught to you, or did you discover them yourself?

Andrew Dalholt: Yes. When I became a 911 dispatcher, at least with my agency, I was taught a lot of stuff, including self stress management. The general education they do is a year long of in-house training. It's very extensive. Then I went for two months to an academy where I lived and did training on site, and that's more for the state. In the in-house training, they teach quite a bit of ways to manage stress.

Jason Michaels: I can imagine that would be very beneficial to your productivity. How long have you been doing this?

Andrew Dalholt: Just over three full years.

Jason Michaels: Have you found that it gets routine or does every day stay unique? While there are always parts of work that become repetitive, does it keep you on your toes a bit?

Andrew Dalholt: Some factors — like entering details about the situation — become routine. Traffic accidents also do, which is about eighty percent of what we do. Then there's the twenty percent that comes in as active calls, which is always different. New elements are always involved, and I have to think quickly on my feet for those. Fortunately, at least three to four times a day we get an active call and are really going at it.

Jason Michaels: So how did you get into this? Did it find you, or did you find it?

Andrew Dalholt: I've always wanted to do something emergency service related, but I couldn't figure out what that was. Then I discovered that I prefer to sit in a chair rather than move around too much. That was a big factor in terms of taking this job. I'm like, "Okay, I get to sit in an office with air conditioning." That sounds pretty nice.

The fact that I am always bouncing around between emergency services — the police side, and the fire department — keeps the work interesting. It's flexible and I get a little bit of each, rather than stay assigned to just one department. When I found this job, I was like, "Why hadn't I thought of this before?" It was a perfect match for everything I wanted to do.

Jason Michaels: That's awesome. When you began your career doing that, was there any element of Tourette's that went into your decision making, or was that not really a part of the equation?

Andrew Dalholt: Not really — because like I said before — a lot of my Tourette's has gone away, and the tics have lessened. When I did have symptoms, I consulted with a medical staff who said there was a possibility that they would start reoccurring in my thirties. Tourette's might become a thing again. I had that in mind when I decided to become a dispatcher and had to ask myself, "If it comes back, is that going to be a problem?" Now that I've done the work, I believe that I could complete my job with the same symptoms I had throughout childhood.

Jason Michaels: I don't know why you wouldn't be able to.

Andrew Dalholt: Exactly. I can't think of anything that would get in the way, mostly because I was fortunate to not have any verbal tics. All of mine were physical. Since the majority of my work involves communications, I wouldn't have any issues. Fortunately, I don't believe that the physical ones would interfere with my position.

Jason Michaels: When Tourette's was more prevalent in your life, did you find it especially challenging?

Andrew Dalholt: I found it annoying.

Jason Michaels: That's a pretty good word for it.

Andrew Dalholt: It was frustrating and annoying, but I never felt like there was anything I couldn't do. It was just that every once in a while

I would get irritated with myself. The thought was more like, ***Dang, I wish this would stop sometimes.*** But I never saw it as a barrier.

Jason Michaels: That's fantastic because sometimes people do see it as prohibiting them from what they want to accomplish. I think it's great that despite the annoyances of the tics, you were able to find something you enjoyed and successfully pursue it. Since you've been doing this job now for three years, you must be doing it well.

When you were younger, were there any hindrances with school such as bullying?

Andrew Dalholt: There were the general hindrances mostly when I was trying to do schoolwork. I'd have my tics and impulses, which would annoy me because they got in the way a bit. I'm sure anyone reading your book who has Tourette's knows it's not the same for everyone, but it's the same idea.

Jason Michaels: What about bullying?

Andrew Dalholt: I didn't deal with much bullying, but mainly because I was very secluded in my school years. I had very few friends, possibly because I was threatened by the idea that I wouldn't feel accepted. For my own personal reasons, I mostly just wanted to be to myself. While I was fortunate to avoid the bullies, that may have occurred because I didn't really talk to anyone in the first place.

Jason Michaels: I understand. Now, let's say a parent, whose child has recently been diagnosed with Tourette syndrome, has picked this book up. They have many questions and wonder how to best support their child. They wonder what their child will be capable of achieving.

In that situation, what would you say to a parent who wants to be the best guide possible as their child navigates Tourette's?

Andrew Dalholt: If they're reading this book, it's clear they already have this in mind. Anyone who seeks out knowledge like this is clearly trying to help their child.

I would say: First, realize if their tics are extensive on a particular day, your child is just as frustrated as you are. After all, they are the ones who are experiencing the tics versus you who simply must deal with them. Focus on creating a calm and accepting atmosphere when this happens. Something that might help you do this is realizing your child doesn't have much choice in the matter. They are probably just as frustrated with the situation as you are.

Jason Michaels: You bring up an interesting point, which is that most people do not understand the rapid, repetitive, unmanageable nature of tics. When you try to explain it to them, their reaction is generally, "What do you mean uncontrollable?"

Andrew Dalholt: Yeah. We don't have a choice because it's an involuntary reaction.

Jason Michaels: That's the perfect response. It took me years to figure out how to explain that unpredictability when I speak to groups. At one point I finally just had to say, "It's not as simple as trying harder to stop the tic because most of the time I don't even know if I'm going to have one." How can you stop something that you aren't aware of in the first place?

Andrew Dalholt: It's like when you have your reflexes tested; when the doctor taps your knee with the reflex hammer, you feel a sensation and have a reaction. It is the same automatic physical response with a tic.

Jason Michaels: Yep. That's great. Let's say that you are talking through the pages of this book to a fifteen-year-old with Tourette's, whose body is changing because of puberty on top of having to deal with uncontrollable tics. What would you say to comfort them so they can get a better grasp on how to handle Tourette's, and how to figure out what they're capable of, and where they want to go in life?

Andrew Dalholt: I'd say watch out for yourself first. This begins with realizing you might not always be able to control your tics. So what if someone else is annoyed by them? If they say, "Don't do that," and your behavior is literally beyond your control, then there is no reason to listen to them. You shouldn't let others get to you.

Jason Michaels: That's so good. I honestly don't know if I've heard anybody give that specific answer before, and I love that. Take care of yourself first. That's fantastic. Is it possible that by dealing with some of the frustrations that come along with Tourette's, you're a stronger person today? I guess we wouldn't know otherwise, because this is just our life. But could you say that there are certain traits that you've developed because of Tourette's?

Andrew Dalholt: I think the independent thinking I've gained from Tourette's goes back to that statement I made earlier about watching out for yourself first. While I would never go out of my way to be an inconvenience to someone, if they are trying to say, "You should do this, that, and the other," I don't respond well to that kind of control. Instead, I'll say, "That's not how I want to live my life because what I really want is X, Y, and Z." In a way, I learned how to live more independently because of Tourette's. When people are always telling you to stop ticcing you start to think, I can't stop so you're just going to have to deal with it. In a way, that lesson of letting go of what other people thought translated into many other parts of my life. If I want to chase a certain dream — or career — and someone says otherwise, I will still always do whatever is best for me.

Jason Michaels: Would you say that mindset has been the most influential in terms of being successful in the direction you went in?

Andrew Dalholt: For sure. Fortunately, my family has always been supportive, yet I never had any chronic fear around my ability to achieve what I wanted. I feel lucky to say that I always believed in myself. For instance, when I was considering leaving my old job, I was heavily discouraged by my colleagues who just didn't want to see me leave. Instead, I said, "I'm going into it anyways." After changing to my current job, I realized I am in a better position because I pursued my passion. Chasing after what you truly want oftentimes leads to a better situation. My life has proven that.

JASON'S SUMMARY

I think it's important to never catastrophize Tourette's because some people are spared from dealing with terrible situations or intense tics. While Andrew certainly dealt with the difficulties and frustrations that come along with Tourette's, he also tried to view them through the lens of an "annoyance." This is a great perspective that keeps things light and has clearly helped him not get bogged down by the condition.

It's also obvious that the training Andrew has done around stress management would benefit anyone living with Tourette's. We not only have to deal with the stress of the tics but also the social stigmas that are sometimes attached to them. Being able to use stress management tools to handle the uncontrollable tics in a healthy way, as well as people's reactions to them, would certainly benefit anyone with Tourette's.

Personally, I find that controlling my breathing helps me manage stressful situations. Especially when I perform on stage, focusing on my breath and the rate of my breathing helps keep me calm, yet alert.

Finally, Andrew's advice that, "You need to watch out for yourself first" is absolute gold. In my resiliency keynote #DoTheImpossible: Resilience, I share how hard it is to take care of others if you aren't taking care of yourself first.

While it can be difficult to stand up for yourself at times, that is exactly what we must do. This comes from a deep understanding that, despite having Tourette's, we are capable of anything we put our minds to. Standing up for your goals, dreams, and viewpoints will speak volumes to those around you. Developing a strong sense of self-respect and boundaries will also help define the way you see yourself.

Allow me to be blunt. If you live with Tourette Syndrome, you are a warrior. Warriors are not victims. While it may sometimes feel as though having Tourette's isn't fair, that is the path that we were given. Stand up fearlessly and unapologetically for yourself and others who might not be as resilient or powerful as you will become. Confidently acting as a warrior will also inspire others to act similarly.

To watch the video of the full interview with Andrew Dalholt, access additional tools to help you live and thrive with Tourette Syndrome, and connect with the Tourette Warrior community, please visit TouretteWarrior.com.

In the next chapter, the interview with Jason Duika, Jason discusses how Tourette Syndrome is inextricably tied to his "musicians' ear" and is one of the reasons he has excelled as a professional opera singer. He also discusses the homeopathic medicines that he still takes to this day and how that, combined with diet and exercise, helped reduce his tics from thousands to virtually none.

CHAPTER 5

JASON DUIKA

OPERA SINGER

Jason Duika is an emerging American Verdi Baritone* who has performed with over ten opera companies across the United States, including Toledo Opera, West Bay Opera, Opera Mississippi, and Palm Beach Opera. He has professionally sung over seventeen operatic roles, including the lead role in Verdi's* Nabucco with West Bay Opera, where critics praised his commanding presence and emotional depth. His return to the Indiana University Jacobs School of Music in 2018 to perform as Enrico in Lucia di Lammermoor was met with acclaim, with critics describing his voice as "manly, generous, and assured." He continued to impress in productions such as La Bohème, I Due Foscari, and Herodiade, and made a notable appearance as a baritone soloist in Vaughan Williams' Dona Nobis Pacem at Carnegie Hall in 2019.

Since the Covid pandemic, Duika has taken on new roles, including Father Germont in La Traviata with West Bay Opera in 2022, Dr. Falke in Die Fledermaus with Opera Mississippi, and Escamillo in Carmen with Boheme Opera of New Jersey, where critics praised his "strong baritone" and "dashing" stage presence. He has also returned to the world-famous Carnegie Hall, performing Mark Hayes' Te Deum with MidAmerica Productions in 2024. A graduate of Alma College, Portland State University, and Indiana University Jacobs School of Music, Duika has honed his craft through young artist programs with Utah Festival Opera, Wichita Grand Opera, and Palm Beach Opera. He now resides in Sylvania, Ohio, and is represented by Randsman Artist Management in New York City while continuing his vocal studies with Andrea DelGiudice.

Jason Michaels: We met at the Tourette Association of America, when they hosted their annual convention in 2022, where you gave an incredible performance. A big group, myself included, gathered around as you performed opera and told your story. I, personally, was blown away by your talent and how successful you had been in the arts. Tell me a bit about what you were like growing up, whether you were curious, outgoing, or quiet.

Jason Duika: I was very curious and outgoing, but I was definitely not quiet. I laugh because when my grandfather and I went shopping — I was six or seven — he was called Molasses, and I was known as Lightning. We'd go shopping as those characters. It would take Molasses six hours to go through one store. And I would've already been in and out of every store within 100 square miles. Hyperactive, hypersensitive, and endlessly curious is how I would describe myself. And I certainly wasn't quiet but rather, verbose. I also was fascinated by science and the world around me. Opera wasn't in my milieu back then, but I did love plate tectonics and marine biology.

For a long time, I wanted to be every profession. People would ask me, "What do you want to be when you grow up?" And I would say, "An architect, a marine biologist, a volcanologist and a doctor." I was inspired, and a lot of that I got from what I like to refer to as "The Tourette."

At this point in my life, I understand how important having the Tourette is to the way in which my brain functions, particularly when it comes to hearing all the different dimensions of music. I sing in nine languages professionally and know I wouldn't have been able to learn them all so quickly were it not for the Tourette. The principal languages I sing in are Italian, French, German, and Russian which I sing in all the time. I've even sung roles by Tchaikovsky, which is in Russian. I also sing a lot in German, French, and Italian and have even performed in Mandarin, Hebrew, Spanish, and Latin. I wouldn't be able to do all of that at such professional speed, or with such alacrity, were it not for the Tourette. Funny to think this all started back then thanks to my insatiable curiosity about the universe.

Jason Michaels: How did the Tourette help you specifically?

Jason Duika: The Tourette has the comorbidity (which means I had several conditions occurring at once). I had what I call the triple cocktail: Tourette Syndrome, ADHD, and OCD. The need for organization and precision, which is a quality that is akin to all of those conditions, is pivotal to being an opera singer. We must sing the most spectacularly difficult music in history for the voice. On top of that, we have to sing the music so precisely according to Strauss, Mozart, or whomever the composer is. That very particular nature lends itself well to the world of opera.

The Tourette, the variation I have is echolalia which means I'm very good at doing accents because I can mimic people. I love people, and people love my accents. Therefore, I do them all the time from German to British. My ability to echo another's voice allowed me to pick up accents easily, similar to language, because of how intensely I listen.

Early on, I realized the Tourette was tied into my musician's ear. I listen to a recording and am able to pick it up rather quickly.

Then I worked very hard over many years to learn how to read music. Now I'm a decent sight-reader, but that's a different skill. I think that the Tourette hampered the learning of the sight-reading, which we all have to be able to do. However, my ear and brain are so inextricably linked to my ability to learn opera now that without the Tourette, I would suffer. The Tourette is such a huge part of my neurology and musician's ears and is what allows me to pick up new material so quickly.

Jason Michaels: Correct me if I'm wrong, but one of the things I talk about in speaking engagements is how living with Tourette's helps you to develop superpowers. It sounds like one of yours is the ability to learn music at a much faster rate than the majority of people.

Jason Duika: Yes. My ability to learn the skeleton of the piece is remarkably quick. Yet I still I have to go back and work very hard to fill in all the little details . Over time, I learned to do a first listen and get it in my ear.

There are people I know in the business who are just blessed with extraordinary abilities. Like the Einsteins of the opera world, they can both sight-read and hear and learn a piece in one sitting.

I have a very special gift to be able to hone in, at least at first blush, listen, and get a lot of what the composer is talking about. And then I have to go back and really be precise.

Jason Michaels: Share with us some of your favorite places that you have performed in your ten years as an opera singer?

Jason Duika: Carnegie Hall was one of them in the big Isaac Stern Auditorium, which seats about 4,000 people.

I had my official professional debut there in June of 2019, before Covid. I sang the baritone solos with MidAmerica Productions performing the famous British composer Vaughn Williams's "Dona Nobis Pacem," which is a sacred piece. Doing this 30-minute piece, which I find so beautiful, alongside 250 other musicians was incredibly special. To top it off, we were in Carnegie Hall, which made the experience even more perfect because of how extraordinary a space it is acoustically.

I have sung two Verdis in my career. I'm a Verdi baritone which, within the opera world, means that my voice type is a specific type of dramatic baritone. Verdi is the famous godfather composer who wrote "La Traviata," which you can hear in the film "Pretty Woman" when Richard Gere takes Julia Roberts to the opera in San Francisco. That's putting it in pop culture sense. Too often, legitimate opera is mistaken for pop opera, or vice versa, which has been defined by talent like Josh Groban, Andrea Bocelli, and Sarah Brightman. The main differentiator is that they use microphones, versus their natural instrument, because their voices are not at the same level of training as mine. My microphone is my body. Legitimate opera singers must project through an orchestra sometimes to the back of a couple thousand-seat auditorium without any amplification. In a sense, we're more like Olympic athletes because of how hard we train.

Jason Michaels: What were some of your favorite performances?

Jason Duika: Some of my favorite performances were the title role in Verdi's Nabucco, which is widely regarded as the heaviest, hardest role in all of Verdi land. That's what devotees call the Verdi repertoire. I performed that role with the West Bay Opera in Palo Alto, California in fall of 2019. It was the last role I did before the Covid pandemic. West Bay Opera is the oldest running opera company behind the San Francisco Opera in the west. It's a very special little gem in Palo Alto, where Stanford is. Those are a couple of my favorites that I've been able to do. I am about to go and sing Dr. Falke in an Operetta, which means "little opera" with Opera Mississippi, a brand-new company. It's always very exciting when you're hired by a new company because it means your career is moving forward. While it's great to be rehired, when a new company wants you, that means you're moving forward. This is my debut with Opera Mississippi, which is the premier opera company in that state. It's a very good company, with a large space in Jackson at Thalia Mara Hall. A lot of famous people have sung there.

I'm the defacto title role Dr. Falke. He doesn't have as much music as the other lead Eisenstein, but it's very fun. The opera, by Johann Strauss II, is called "Die Fledermaus," which means revenge of the bat. An operetta is more akin to a play meaning the performers have dialogue and we also sing.

So that's what I'm about to do. Then I'll be making my debut in another opera here with Toledo Opera where I live in Toledo, Ohio, which is another great company.

Unfortunately, the nature of the business means that I have made a living out of auditioning. I am constantly forced to put myself out there even though I have been successful in other operas and sung at a number of venues. It's just how the industry operates.

Jason Michaels: You have been able to do something that was a dream of yours for a while. Yet, at what point did you fall in love with it?

Jason Duika: In my late teens I wanted to be a pop singer or a jazz singer. Those were my favorite types of music at the time. But I always had a more naturally operatic sound, because that's how I had been trained with voice lessons. Sadly, opera singers in their early twenties do not exist. There barely begins to be an opera singer at twenty-five, because of the maturation of the voice.

When I attended Alma College, a private liberal arts school in Michigan, I had an English professor my freshman year who, along with her husband, was a classical music fan. She said to me one day, "You should sing opera." I was eighteen at the time so I was perplexed. My reaction was, "Opera?" but she ended up being right! I started to visit the library and check out opera recordings. From there, I decided to sing in the school choir and take voice lessons. Once opera found me, I fell in love with it.

I think if I were to go back, I would warn my twenty-year-old self just how much work is involved. There is indeed a lot of sacrifice because opera really is one of the hardest things to do in the world. Even after you have earned multiple degrees, completed young artist programs, considered journeyman professional-level extensions of your education, and acquired a manager, you can still end up with absolutely nothing.

Opera is far from a secure paycheck or lifestyle. Yet, it's one of the most demanding jobs that I can think of. Either Businessweek or Newsweek ran an article some years ago stating opera singer as one of the most difficult jobs in the world.

Jason Michaels: What advice do you share with young opera singers?

Jason Duika: I have a private studio of young voice students — some of whom are singing professionally — that I encourage. The work is very meaningful to me. I often tell them, "Don't pursue this unless it wakes you up in the middle of the night, it's the last thing you think about before you go to bed, the first thing you think about in the morning."

As I tell my students, "You cut me, I bleed opera. It's the reason God put me here on earth. Don't pursue it unless that's how you feel, too, because it will take everything and give nothing back. There are great years where you're singing all over the place, and lean years where you get one contract. And you can be successful, but it is a war of attrition." Anyway, that's a topic for another time.

Jason Michaels: It's very true. Being an entertainer, I understand the struggle. Going back to when you were younger, do you remember recognizing that there was something going on regarding tics?

Jason Duika: I don't remember it, but my mother does. She's told me many times about an incident I had at age five and a half when we were outside walking. My feet turned inwards, and I just couldn't stop them from doing that. She wanted to know what that was, as any prudent parent would. From there, we went to the doctor, and I was diagnosed with Tourette Syndrome just shy of age six. Within a year, I had a huge variety of tics. Unfortunately, the condition kept progressing because by the time I was twelve, I had a world-class case.

We went to the Mayo Clinic, and finally the Henry Ford Hospital, where the physicians said it was the most severe case they had ever seen. I had whiplash tic seizures that were so bad my mom had to hold me down on the floor during piano lessons so I wouldn't snap my own neck. To alleviate that tic, they tried injecting botulinum toxin with a huge needle into my neck to numb that area. This instead resulted in the most excruciating pain and was so scary. I also had Echolalia and Copropraxia. I had everything.

Then there was also the fact that I was constantly made fun of. I am forty this year, and twenty-something years ago Tourette's didn't have the same level of understanding that it does now. This is even in comparison with autism, which shares the same gene, and at least had national awareness commercials. For those that don't know — autism, Tourette's, OCD, and AHDH are all on the same gene. Yet neurodivergency was not widely understood, and so many people thought I was creating the behavior myself, making it up, having fun. Being ostracized by everyone around me resulted in feeling like I had a giant scarlet "T" on my back. I mean, I was just beaten up. When I was twelve or thirteen, students took turns holding me down in the back of the bus and spitting on me. There was that abuse, which included many more moments, on top of the actual Tourette's symptoms to deal with.

Jason Michaels: How did that impact your physical and mental health?

Jason Duika: I never tried to commit suicide, but I was at the end of my rope as any human would be. When any human reaches that level of stress, they have goofy thoughts about dying to ease the tremendous unending nature of it. ***Is this going to be the way life is forever?*** I used to wonder. Talk about stress-inducing.

Through diet, exercise, and a relentless pursuit of knowledge by my mother, we found what we call a "cure." While I don't know if one truly exists, I diffused my Tourette's to livable levels. I made it mine and never looked back. Yet, twenty-something years later, I still struggle with the mental aspect of the condition a lot, which includes anxiety and obsessive thoughts. I worry a lot about my voice and career.

Jason Michaels: Similar to you, who had your mother as a champion, I also had my parents who were my support group. As awful as it is, how you deal with being ostracized and bullied is all about perspective. Yet that is hard to have at age thirteen when people are beating you up because of behavior they don't understand. On the flip side, as you said, we live in a different world today where there is a great deal more education. Unfortunately, that doesn't mean everybody's going to treat you right, and, in a way, we are lucky to be prepared to deal with adversity so gracefully. When you face it as an adult, you are already prepared how to handle it. How did your teachers react?

Jason Duika: I was blessed in the respect that most of my teachers were really lovely, thoughtful, and understanding. They were patient for the most part and found extracurricular ways to help me, especially when it came to standardized testing which is such a misnomer. Even people who are not neurodivergent have struggled with standardized testing. It's crappy for most people. Fortunately, they know a lot more about it now, and they found ways back then to give me quizzes or tests orally. I knew the information and would score very high, yet had to do it in my own way. Still, mathematics was always difficult. I never really had a brain for numbers.

However, oddly enough, my brain understands the surreal number chart*, which includes numbers that are based on 10. It reminds me of that savant-like ability that most people with Tourette's have. Higher math — which included Geometry, Algebra 2, and Calculus — I skipped because it was beyond the way my brain understood numbers. Yet conversely, my brain understands the music of math so beautifully.

It's a curious thing, the brain. Then you add Tourette's, or whatever neurodivergent condition you want, and get a more complicated palette from which to paint the world. Naturally, this influences what the world represents to you. So, fortunately I had teachers who honored this by finding ways to help me retain information and then tested me appropriately. It certainly took some creative thinking on their part. This extraordinary set of teachers that I was blessed with are still some of my dear friends today because of how they let me be creative, explore, and try new things.

While college was a lot more difficult, my teachers were equally as understanding. Thankfully, by then the physical nature of Tourette's had retreated to my brain* because by my seventeenth or eighteenth year we noticed an eighty-something percentile reduction in tics.

Jason Michaels: Wow.

Jason Duika: This happened when we found the proper diet and proper supplements. When I was young, the doctors shoved Anafranil* at me. It made the Tourette ten times worse. So, we got me off all that crap. And I tend to be weary of allopathy*. I tend to do a lot of homeopathy*, even to this day. The only thing I am on today is ten milligrams of an anti-anxiety medication. I take a couple at night to help me sleep and deal with being an adult in a more turbulent world, and an opera singer at that. As glamorous as being an opera singer can be, I never know where my next paycheck will come from. It's also so much work.

Getting back to homeopathy, a practice I still follow, that was the cocktail that allowed me to overcome — and I use that word lightly so no one takes offense — my tics. Essentially, it made them livable because they dropped from thousands in a day to dozens and finally, none. By the time I arrived at college, the slate was wiped clean. I could finally be myself.

Jason Michaels: Wow. Were there any other miracles that happened thanks to the Tourette?

Jason Duika: In spite of the Tourette, I was known for my singing voice, physique, and intellect. In a way, as I've realized recently, it probably saved me from making a lot of early mistakes like other people in their teen years. Yet I still came into my own a lot later in life, around my mid-twenties instead of age fifteen or sixteen. There were definitely some delayed gratification, Cinderella-story elements to that period because I blossomed so much later than most. Thankfully, now I look back on that as totally okay.

Jason Michaels: Above all, who was most critical to helping you during the most challenging times with your Tourette's?

Jason Duika: I had extraordinary teachers in college who are still dear friends to this day and have actually traveled to hear me sing. Yet, I was incredibly blessed to have the most supportive parents who are truly the rock from which I am built. Neurodivergent children need overly understanding parents who are never willing to give up on them. To not have that is just criminal in my opinion. My mother just never gave up, and I am still very grateful to her.

Jason Michaels: If you had to summarize what your high school teachers did for you, what would you say?

Jason Duika: All of my teachers in the collegiate and high school realms were beyond patient and willing to go to any lengths to help me absorb and retain information. Above all, I am grateful for the environment they created in which I felt safe.

I taught high school as I was building my opera career as of five or six years ago. That work environment taught me how to heal from my own horrible high school experience with my peers. Being the opera substitute for six years, I had a completely disparate experience as I was very popular. Some of those students are still dear friends of mine. That moment in time taught me a lot about humanity and humility. I didn't make much financially so I had to give it up eventually. The hours were terrible, the days were atrociously long, and I was always sick.

Jason Michaels: You mentioned that diet and exercise played a huge part in reducing your tics. For instance, I still drink coffee but know it is better for me to not indulge in caffeine since it is frequently linked to increased motor and vocal tics. What did you figure out that worked for you?

Jason Duika: My wellness plan has changed so much over the last twenty years. I've realized that my diet should be gluten-free or, at the very least, I should be mindful of not indulging in enriched doughs like croissants, bagels, and donuts. Things of that nature seem to affect my Tourette's. Sugar should also be kept at a minimum. Most importantly, I engage in regular exercise and have been a gym rat and an amateur bodybuilder for the last twenty years. I practically live at the gym, which makes me feel less tense, anxious, and more readily able to face the difficulties of this tumultuous world that we live in. In every way, shape, and form, it helps me mentally handle wars and all the current affairs we have to process every day.

Jason Michaels: Let me interrupt you because I also spend a lot of time in the gym as well. So, you're talking about the physical benefits of exercise, but do you also find that it helps with the mental components of Tourette's, because I do. I find that it's tremendously —

Jason Duika: Inextricably linked.

I did TaeKwonDo for five years and made it all the way to my black belt. It gave me a tremendous sense of purpose to be within that team who I felt accepted me. The interesting thing was that I wouldn't tic when I was doing these sequences of movements, the way that my teachers taught them. Those mindfulness practices and disciplines, which are the essential nature of the dedicated Korean forms, still help me very much. I practiced Taekwondo for years because I found exertion of the body calms the mind, releases endorphins, and sweat of course. That exertion has been profound in terms of me handling Tourette's.

Being mindful of maintaining a holistic diet also helps. I found homeopathy through a company that produces a sleep aid with valerian root, which I still take a few of at bedtime. When I do a huge performance, especially when I travel, I take one under the tongue, and it calms my nerves naturally. It was a delicate balance between maintaining my mental and spiritual sides. While I'm not religious, I do believe in God, who I see as the creator of the universe. The way in which diet and exercise intersected to alleviate my Tourette's was tremendously spiritual for me. Plus, fortunately, post-puberty my brain chemistry finally settled down and helped me to create a more calming environment so I could live a "normal" life — whatever that is.

Jason Michaels: You mentioned that when you were executing the TaeKwonDo forms that you had no tics. I just call it a level of focus. You're just completely consumed with what you're doing at the moment. Is this also true when you are on stage?

Jason Duika: Yes. Unquestionably. I tic a little before I go out on stage, but once I become the character they go away. It's a remarkable thing. I am what I refer to as a singing actor; and the number of lines I have to deliver, my breath which I have to focus on, and the orchestra's music is all very transportive.

You get to a point professionally, and this is said with the greatest amount of humility, where you amaze yourself. It is incredible that your body can create such an extraordinary sound that can carry over a huge orchestra to the back of a full house. However, I always remind myself that none of this would be possible without Tourette's and the degree to which it has affected my brain and ear. Ironically, once you arrive onstage after doing all the work, none of that even matters. It's as if there is no Tourette's or boundaries. It's just your own voice, the music, and the sound blending together. Of course, it's also about interacting with your co-stars as well.

Jason Michaels: I'll just ask for clarification, but would you say to a certain extent that, despite the difficulties you faced as an adolescent, Tourette's has empowered you?

Jason Duika: Yes, unquestionably so. I wouldn't be who I am without it but, I also would never want it to dominate my life again. Fortunately, I don't think that type of control is going to return.

Jason Michaels: It sounds like you now have a certain level of life experience that you can draw on to live more peacefully in your own body. While Tourette Syndrome is an extremely serious disorder, are there any funny stories that resulted because of your condition?

Jason Duika: Yes! One day, when I was in school, I was in an assembly alongside hundreds of other kids. I started having a swearing fit, which of course led to the other kids egging me on. While I was doing my best to stop this behavior, the harder I tried, the more I had to do it. So, I just blurted out a plethora of "fuck, ass, tits," or whatever other profanities came out of my mouth. It was an earful, that's for sure, and one I fortunately don't remember. My counselor, who reminded me of the actress Susan Lucci from the soap "Days of Our Lives," was also there. Over and over, I said, "Susan Lucci!" even though that clearly wasn't her real name. Everyone, including the administration, just lost it. When they came over to check on me, I couldn't stop laughing and said, "I'm sorry, but I couldn't hold it in anymore!" Thankfully, their response was, "That's okay" because everyone thought it was hilarious.

Jason Michaels: Is there anything else you want to share about living with Tourette's, or about the condition in general?

Jason Duika: We are all on our own journey. We all have our own struggles. On top of that, there is an enormous self-imposed pressure people with Tourette's put on themselves not to tic. Outwardly, from the point of view of others, it might even seem like we can help ourselves, but we can't. Those two combined create even more internal pressure to do it. So, we don't need the world's opinions. After years of that pressure, which often sounded like ***Stay in your lane, don't make a sound, don't tic, and certainly don't swear,*** I was like a little volcano a lot of the time. This is because I was trying so hard. You realize that while pressure still exists today it is totally sublimated and disparate. I would tell the world to manage, rather than lower, your expectations of how we are supposed to act.

While not intended to be self-aggrandizing, I want to be a beacon for the Tourette community and say, "Look what a Touretter can become. Look what we can do." I knew that in order to achieve a "normal" life, which means many things to different people, it would come down to working on myself.

The world tends to embrace these types of stories, but it also tends to be very hostile to talent. Since we met at the Tourette Association, I had my main stage audition for the largest, most important opera company on the planet, the Metropolitan Opera. I'm waiting right now to see where I fit in their next season. So, talk about pins and needles.

It's one of the most storied houses in the world made even more famous by "The Met: Live in HD," which is their award-winning series that has brought live performances to movie theaters for years. So, look at what someone like myself can accomplish when they're not antagonized or pre-judged. If you are given respect and the space to be calm, just like a cancer patient or someone who is autistic, you can do incredible things. Thankfully, our community now has the world-famous Billie Eilish who is openly talking about her own struggle with Tourette's. The hope is that publicity will lead to a greater understanding of Tourette's and respect for those of us who have it.

Jason Michaels: I know what it's like to be a child with Tourette Syndrome, but I imagine it was pretty terrifying to be my parents, too. Considering most parents want the best for their children, what do you tell one whose kid has just been told, "You have Tourette's and there's not a damn thing you can do about it"?

Jason Duika: It all comes down to knowledge and acceptance. I once had a student who had Tourette's, but his parents refused to accept it. Following their lead, so did he. On top of it, he was abusive and nasty. One time when I was substitute teaching, I tried to talk to him after which he swore at me. The authorities had to take him down to their offices after his outburst. It was unfortunate because all I kept saying was, "Because I have Tourette's, I can help you understand your condition and how to learn to live with it." The way his parents refused to acknowledge his condition is the absolute worst thing you can do. They pretended like it wasn't real, which will always blow up in someone's face. Not that I would wish any harm on them, but their refusal to see what was real is not the way to deal with Tourette's.

Jason Michaels: It took me a long time to feel comfortable talking about Tourette's; but once I did start, it was incredibly healing. Still, there's no question that connection between openness and acceptance was surprising to me. I didn't see it coming.

Jason Duika: That makes sense. However, in the circumstances of that student and his parents, they just swept it under the rug. Then on top of that, the parents were nasty and defensive, and the student abusive. All I kept thinking after he tried to get physical with me was: ***After high school, this is going to go further south so I would find a way right now for you and your parents to come together and accept your Tourette's.*** They were in a unique position to work with someone who had overcome it as an adult. I could have helped them cope in a healthy manner, but that may have ticked him off even more. All that being said, acceptance around any condition is always key as that is the only place from which you can learn about it. You aren't going to get anywhere from a place of panic. Instead, the attitude should be — whether it's a mild or severe case — let's discover what this is because we don't know all of the details yet. You must take it day by day.

Jason Michaels: So, is that your message to parents?

Jason Duika: And to see what gifts can come out of it.

Jason Michaels: I agree with you 100% since that is where I am at this point of life. When I talk to groups about overcoming difficult situations, I often say, "What may seem impossible to deal with, or so overwhelming, might ultimately define you. It could one day even be seen as a gift." Yet, that seems like a crazy idea when you feel like you're being tortured.

So getting back to your advice, how would you approach a thirteen-year-old who is ticcing like crazy and feels like this persecution will never end? What do you say to that person?

Jason Duika: Seek inspiration. Realize you were put on this earth for a purpose that goes beyond Tourette's. I'll say it again for emphasis: seek inspiration.

Jason Michaels: Hey. You're going to make me emotional here.

Jason Duika: Seek out something that will allow your talents and gifts to betray a single purpose. Choose an activity that will reveal your deeper meaning, whatever that might be. For example, at the same conference where I met you, I also connected with a young artist whose extraordinary gifts lie in painting murals. The good news is that Touretters tend to be highly intelligent. In addition to that, they are also atypically articulate and tend to have savant-like gifts. My incredible gift manifested in music, but others might draw, write, act, or communicate in a different way.

I always think back on how my parents encouraged me to be open about my condition. They even had a t-shirt made, which I would wear on flights because they turned out to be particularly difficult. On one flight to Florida, when I was twelve or thirteen, my mom counted something crazy like 1,400 tics of every kind imaginable. Yet this t-shirt that I always wore — which said, "I have Tourette Syndrome, I can't help it" — opened doors because it had an explanation of the condition on the back. That would precipitate conversation and a paradigm shift. The sense of self-advocacy which my parents instilled in me, even prior to Tourette's becoming public knowledge, really boosted my self-confidence. Perhaps it is why I always go back to the advice, "Seek inspiration."

Jason Michaels: It's wonderful. I want to ask one more question because the inspiration behind this whole project is to honor people who have had success while having to live with and handle all the challenges of Tourette's. So, if you had to boil it down to a couple of things, what would you attribute your success to?

Jason Duika: I've always been a relentless perseverer, which isn't a word.

Jason Michaels: It's a good enough word for now.

Jason Duika: My perseverance has been relentless. I always knew that I had a destiny that went beyond struggling with Tourette's. Yet, it took me a long time to realize that. A hairstylist who I worked with at my first professional gig eleven years ago made a huge impact on deciding to be more open about my story. One day before I went out on stage at the Utah Festival Opera she said to me, "You need not keep your struggle a secret, but rather share it with people." Almost fortuitously, the following year I was asked to give the 2013 Distinguished Alumni Address at my old high school's graduation. This was at the Hill Auditorium at the University of Michigan, and I spoke in front of 4,500 people. It was the first time my parents helped me write this story, and I cried through the whole thing. Afterwards, I got a standing ovation before I sang, after which I received another one. In that moment, I realized it was necessary for me to start finding different outlets to talk about my experience. However, I was still terrified in that moment because I didn't know what response I was going to receive. I realized that it was necessary for me to start sharing. So, I found different ways to do that. I didn't know what kind of response I was going to get. I was terrified. But I always knew I had a destiny.

In high school I was known as "The Tourette's Kid," which certainly wasn't meant as a compliment. I felt absolute revulsion when I realized that was my nickname. So, looking back at how far I have come, I believe that growth cycles back to two things: relentless perseverance and the notion that I had a destiny. Today, after many years of feeling silenced, I feel like the poster child for neurodivergency and anyone without a voice.

JASON'S SUMMARY

Jason's willingness to be so open and honest about his journey living with Tourette's is inspiring.

The first thing that I took note of in our conversation was that Jason actively used the comorbidities that often accompany Tourette's as a strength instead of a weakness. He viewed the traits that went along with these co-occuring conditions, like OCD and ADHD, as helpful.

Let's review some of the things he said that explained how he uses characteristics which are oftentimes looked down upon to lift him up professionally. In Jason's own words: "Tourette Syndrome, ADHD, and OCD. The need for organization and precision, which is a quality that is akin to all of those conditions, is pivotal to being an opera singer."

He also said: "I realized the Tourette was tied into my musician's ear. I listen to a recording and am able to pick it up rather quickly." And, "My ear and brain are so inextricably linked to my ability to learn opera now that without the Tourette, I would suffer. Tourette's is such a huge part of my neurology and musician's ear and is what allows me to pick up new material so quickly."

At another point in the interview Jason made this comment about the way he viewed the tics initially before he found peace with them, "Is this going to be the way life is forever?"

I, too, felt that way when I was living through the most pronounced times of my tics. I think all of us who have gone through violent levels of them have had similar sentiments. My point is that it is normal to feel like tics might be never-ending at certain moments in life. Honestly, my very best advice to anyone struggling with tics is to find a friend, family member, or medical professional to express your frustrations to. Also, please realize that it is normal and understandable to feel anger. Expressing any emotions that cause distress, rather than bottling them up, will help you manage your tics so much better.

It may be difficult to understand, but at this point in my life, I have simply accepted that certain chapters will be full of tics. Being okay with that has made a tremendous difference in my quality of life. On the other hand, you can also look through the lens of having to deal with tics all day long as unbearable. Yes, you might feel like you are being tortured at times; but truly, it is all a matter of perspective. At some point, I simply accepted that tics are a normal part of my life and stopped thinking about them completely. Today, I choose to live with them. After all, what you resist persists.

Jason's insights into diet and exercise are worth special consideration for how to manage both tics and mental health. While this is not a medical journal, nor should Jason's answer be construed as medical advice, his insights into the benefits of homeopathy are eye-opening.

He explained the adjoining psychological and physical approach that was taken to alleviate his Tourette's when he said, "Through diet, exercise, and a relentless pursuit of knowledge by my mother, we found what we call 'a cure.' While I don't know if one truly exists, I diffused my Tourette's to livable levels. I made it mine and never looked back."

He also said, "I tend to do a lot of homeopathy, even to this day."

And, "That was the cocktail that allowed me to overcome — and I use that word lightly so no one takes offense — my tics. Essentially, it made them livable because they dropped from thousands in a day to dozens and finally, none. By the time I got to college, the slate was wiped clean. I could finally be myself."

Jason also shared how much exercise helps him. He said, "I practically live at the gym, which makes me feel less tense, anxious, and more readily able to face the difficulties of this tumultuous world we live in." And, "I found exertion of the body calms the mind, releases endorphins, and sweat of course. That exertion has been profound in terms of me handling Tourette's. Being mindful of maintaining a holistic diet also helps."

Honestly, there's not a lot more to say, other than what Jason articulated. Personally, exercise has helped me manage my physical and mental health in a safe, natural manner. I highly recommend it for anyone that is struggling with tics.

Jason's relationship with his teachers and how they worked with him, particularly when it came to his auditory learning style, was worthy of note, "I was blessed in the respect that most of my teachers were really lovely, thoughtful, and understanding. They were patient for the most part and found extracurricular ways to help me, especially when it came to standardized testing which is such a misnomer. Even people who are not neurodivergent have struggled with standardized testing. They found ways back then to give me quizzes or tests orally. I knew the information and would score very high."

I wonder if you can learn from Jason's example and advocate for yourself or your loved one if there is a struggle with testing in school. Intelligence has nothing to do with testing well. It simply means that you don't test well in a very specific manner. As Jason mentioned above, there are many ways that someone can be tested. Perhaps, you simply need a different method.

When Jason brought up how his parents supported him, I felt as though that deserved more attention. It should be noted that when people are put in situations where they feel safe, they thrive. Here is what he said, "I was incredibly blessed to have the most supportive parents who are truly the rock from which I am built. Neurodivergent children need overly understanding parents who are willing to never give up on them. To not have that is just criminal in my opinion. My mother just never gave up, and I am still very grateful to her."

Jason also felt supported by his teachers. He said, "All my teachers in the collegiate and high school realms were beyond patient and willing to go to any lengths to help me absorb and retain the information. Above all, I am grateful for the environment they created in which I felt safe."

It is powerful that Jason said the word "safe" to further emphasize the impact this has on someone's ability to succeed. When we feel seen, heard, acknowledged, and supported, we are better able to handle the difficulties of living with tics. Then, we can calmly and confidently find the things that we are passionate about.

Above all, isn't Jason's passion for opera inspiring? Passion is the one word I would use to describe this interview. Jason's deep love, respect, and adoration for opera can literally be felt through the words on these pages. He is an example of someone who found his passion, and he challenges us when he says, "Seek inspiration. Realize you were put on this earth for a purpose that goes beyond Tourette's. I'll say it again for emphasis: seek inspiration."

He reminds us: "Touretters tend to be highly intelligent. In addition to that, they are also atypically articulate and tend to have savant-like gifts."

Jason continued to explain, "My incredible gift manifested in music, but others might draw, write, act, or communicate in a different way."

It's important to note that those of us who live with Tourette Syndrome have incredible abilities that other, "normal" people may not have. We have superpowers that are forged through the fire of living with tics. Ask yourself this question, "What inspires me? What do I love deeply?"

Don't worry if there isn't an immediate answer to this question. Just by asking the question, your brain will seek to find an answer. I've had answers come long after I posed an inquiry. The key is to be searching for the answer and open to it.

The final thing that I wanted to point out was Jason's realization that educating others through his own narrative was an important moment of growth. He said, "I realized that it was necessary for me to start sharing. So, I found different ways to do that. I didn't know what kind of response I was going to get. I was terrified. But I always knew I had a destiny."

Personally, I had no interest in talking about Tourette's or educating anyone until I was in my mid-thirties. Once I started speaking about it and sharing my story, I was shocked by how healing it was. I agree with Jason's comment. Helping Touretters and their families and friends has been life changing.

---

*A Verdi Baritone is an elite, dramatic voice type characterized by a rich, powerful tone, high tessitura comfort, and immense stamina, essential for lead roles. (Wikipedia)

*Giuseppe Verdi was an Italian composer best known for his operas. (Wikipedia)

* In mathematics, the surreal number system is a totally ordered proper class containing not only the real numbers but also infinite and infinitesimal numbers, respectively larger or smaller in absolute value than any positive real number. (Wikipedia)

*When Jason said "retreated to my brain" he was referring to how tics can be internalized as thoughts rather than externalized as actions.

*Anafranil is a tricyclic antidepressant (TCA) primarily used to treat Obsessive-Compulsive Disorder (OCD) in adults and children. It works by increasing serotonin and norepinephrine levels in the brain.

*Allopathy, or allopathic medicine, refers to conventional, evidence-based medical practice that treats diseases through methods opposing the symptoms, such as pharmaceutical drugs, surgery, or radiation. It is commonly known as Western, mainstream, or modern medicine. (Google)

*Homeopathy is a system of alternative medicine developed in 1796 by Samuel Hahnemann, based on the principles of "like cures like" (treating symptoms with substances that cause similar symptoms) and extreme dilution. It uses highly diluted substances from plants, minerals, or animals to treat. (Google)

To watch the video of the full interview with Jason Duika, access additional tools to help you live and thrive with Tourette Syndrome, and connect with the Tourette Warrior community, please visit TouretteWarrior.com.

In the next chapter, the interview with Jacob Weiss, Jacob discusses some of the sensory aspects of living with Tourette's. He also shares that he believes that the way people approach creativity and academic work is similar to the way that people with Tourette's and OCD think.

CHAPTER 6

JACOB WEISS

EXECUTIVE DIRECTOR OF PLAYING BY AIR

Jacob Weiss, PhD, is the founder of Hand Eye Body Academy, a virtual social enterprise. His mission is to help people move, focus, and function with more ease by teaching hand-eye coordination exercises. Creative, fun, and accessible for all abilities, Jacob has taken his expertise in hand-eye coordination skills to help people around the world, thanks to the web.

As the Executive Director of Playing By Air, a theatrical performance troupe, Jacob grew his childhood passion for juggling into an acclaimed touring program that makes a difference for organizations, families, and communities around the world by donating a performance for hospitals, schools, and nonprofits for every gig they book. Playing By Air specializes in juggling choreography which includes elements of dance, movement, and showmanship in their performances. Impressively, this troupe has performed at the White House and in front of 20,000 people at Madison Square Garden.

In spite of his science background — having earned a PhD at Vanderbilt University in Biomedical Informatics after graduating from Princeton — the brilliant Dr. Weiss has had the greatest impact as an entertainer. By marrying his academic brain and highly acclaimed performance skills, he has developed interactive training programs and touring shows that have helped teachers, trainers, coaches, therapists, movement educators, and organizations around the world.

Jason Michaels: Jacob, you're someone I've known for quite some time, but the reader might be unfamiliar with your impressive background. Tell us the short version of who you are and what you do.

Jacob Weiss: I currently run a program that is centered on training teachers and coaches in hand-eye coordination and movement training. I also have been a professional juggler for over a decade now. My company, Hand Eye Body, weaves together my background in PhD research work in online community building and resources, which is essentially geared towards designing virtual tools for health and wellness.

Jason Michaels: Not only are you very well established, but you are also a high performer. You understand how to commit to something and see it all the way through, which I admire. I love that because I think it is an important lesson for us all. Were you always this way?

Jacob Weiss: One trait that crosses over to my childhood is that I had a lot of energy as a kid. I started playing basketball and dribbling around the court when I was three years old, and its been a part of my life ever since — even before I learned how to juggle at age ten, long before I was able to spin a basketball on my finger. I was always trying to learn something new and took a very playful approach to it. In many ways, I was a mix of silly and outgoing but also had a reserved side to my personality. I could be shy or quiet at times.

I got diagnosed with Tourette's when I was ten. I feel very lucky in respect that juggling — which is in a sense like a moving meditation — helped me manage my condition. By juggling for a few hours outdoors after school, all my energy was able to flow through.

Jason Michaels: Was there an element of you being a "performer" when you were young?

Jacob Weiss: Apparently, when I was about four, I was singing "It's a Small World" with a group of kids, and I jumped out from the group and started dancing around.

I've always been interested in Vaudeville and physical comedy and that kind of thing. I wasn't into traditional singing or the theater-type of performing, which were probably too serious for me. Instead, I would always be doing tricks, like spinning the basketball at basketball camp when I was six years old. Even early on I attracted attention, as I remember being interviewed by the TV station who was doing a story on our camp. So I had an element of performer in me, but it wasn't the traditional-type, but rather about showmanship of performing.

Jason Michaels: When do you remember having tics show up?

Jacob Weiss: The sensory aspects of Tourette's and OCD can blend together because that sensitivity and "right now" feeling where you must get your energy out is very similar. However, I remember having my first Tourette's tics at age four, five, and six. The first indication of it was how long it would take me to pick out a pair of socks that didn't scratch my feet. I'd have to go through a bunch of pairs to find one that wouldn't bother me. Some early tics were eye blinking and throat clearing. Then I went through a period where I would spit, which was not fun for my parents. My mom's field of work is around medical diagnosis, so fortunately, she studied Tourette's and diagnosed me herself. Then we went into a traditional physician's office, and I was officially diagnosed with Tourette's around ten years old.

Jason Michaels: What was it like for the people that you surrounded yourself with? Obviously, I'm talking about immediate family, but I'm also referring to your friends and schoolmates. This might be a little bit too broad; but as a general rule, were people supportive of you? As you remember back on that time, how did you feel?

Jacob Weiss: My parents and family were really supportive, so I didn't feel the need to participate in Tourette support groups while growing up. My parents were very understanding and patient. I think that patience is one of the key words there. My close friends were also nice and supportive. Yet, as we all know, in school there are close and then looser friends. The latter could be nice but also blend in with the bullying crowd.

There were definitely some aspects of teasing. Around fifth or sixth grade, I remember one kid figuring out that a gesture he made set off a tic where I had to shake my head violently back and forth. When he figured that out, instead of stopping, he kept doing it throughout class.

Jason Michaels: That's terrible.

Jacob Weiss: That was not the most fun time. Overall though, people were pretty supportive. My teachers tried their best but didn't always understand. Sometimes they thought I was intentionally trying to be disruptive, like when I would tap my notebook on the desk repeatedly. They scolded me to stop doing that instead of doing further investigation. Even if they understood that the eye blinking or throat clearing were part of Tourette's, they weren't always aware of certain actions that were mixed in as well.

Jason Michaels: I find it so interesting because I've read countless stories of people whose teachers have bullied them. I find that shocking and infuriating. I know that we Touretters can get on people's nerves if they don't completely understand what we're doing. Our behavior can certainly test people. I just find it problematic when people who are supposed to be there to support us end up making life harder.

Jacob Weiss: I never thought of it as bullying. The way I saw it was more that they didn't understand the extent of Tourette's in terms of the many forms it can take on. If they're not living with it, it's easy to misunderstand and hard to tell what a tic is. It's especially difficult when the child is silly to begin with because you don't know if they are just playing around. It's a fine line and can be a challenge for someone on the outside to know.

Jason Michaels: That's fair. Obviously, you and I, and most people with Tourette's, know that the tics wax and wane. Sometimes they're severe, and sometimes they're not. If you had to classify your level of severity on a sliding scale, what did it feel like to you? Between one and ten, with one being the lighter side and ten representing severe, where do you feel your tics fell?

Jacob Weiss: It's a wide range between three and eight. Fortunately, my tics were never so extreme that they were physically debilitating. There were times, maybe an hour, when I was incapacitated, but it didn't stop me from doing what I wanted to do. There were times when life was more stressful, such as final exam times, and that could make the tics worse. Yet the tics became more subtle over time. As I reached my late high school years and then college, I would hold my breath or flex my jaw, which were less visible tics than my other tics. Then there would be times that I would hold the tics back, meaning they were worse when I got home. Even as an adult, particularly when I am performing or speaking, I still have to tic the second I exit stage left. On stage there are no tics because I am in that zone of flow. Yet, when I arrive backstage, or am in the dressing room, I'll be zipping and unzipping my suitcase repeatedly. Then if I get comfortable, I'll blink my eyes more. It's amazing how when I am in presenting or performing mode, which I know many Touretters can relate to, any inclinations to tic are completely gone.

Jason Michaels: I find myself chuckling at how insanely familiar what you're talking about is. Every example has me thinking, *I do that too.* So, if I understand correctly, you go into a hyper-focused zone when performing that is a bit different than everyday life. Almost putting a bubble around your psyche must push away the tics.

Let's talk about everyday life. How did you or do you deal with the tics? Do you try to mask them in another movement? Do you try to hide them so people at the grocery store won't freak out. Or was it more like, ***You know what? I'm just going to tell the world. If they're going to see it anyways, I might as well be the one to let them know.***

Jacob Weiss: Sometimes I would try to hide them and then other times I wouldn't. Or I would try to blend them in with other things I was doing. For instance, if I had to make a "T" sound I could satisfy that urge by phrasing my sentences so they included a "T." That would stop me from repeating the "T" sound. Or, if I absolutely had to repeat something, I would do it in a way where reiterating a certain word made me seem thoughtful.

Jason Michaels: That makes perfect sense.

Jacob Weiss: I probably still implement some of those tactics. While I haven't in recent years, when I was in high school and a bit older, I would mask the urge to repeat a word by making it seem as though I was asking a question. By phrasing that same word in a slightly different way I could stop myself from ticcing.

Jason Michaels: That's fascinating.

Jacob Weiss: There were other ways to weave my tics into everyday life. Once, I was eating a snack or lunch, and for whatever reason, sniffing my food became my tic. Blowing out through my mouth as I was eating the food is how I satisfied it. One of the other kids was like, "Why are you smelling your food before you eat it?" which was pretty funny even to me. That is an example of where I wouldn't try to hide the tic, but there were other times where it was easier to hold back and then allow it to come out at home.

Jason Michaels: Can you recall ever having a situation where you were not able to do or accomplish something due to your Tourette's? Or a time where somebody closed a door on you, or you couldn't participate in a certain opportunity because of it?

Jacob Weiss: Not that I can think of. If anything, being separated from others could be helpful, like when I was asked to take standardized testing in my own room. Prior to this, I took my regular exams at a big table with six other students at it. Thanks to the stress, I started ticcing by hitting my hand on the table. Shaking the table so forcefully made the exams even more stressful for everyone involved. Fortunately, I started taking those standardized exams in a separate room with a glass window, which made it feel like I was in the same space with everyone else even though I was separate. That was very accommodating to my Tourette's.

Jason Michaels: That's great. If you were to educate the world about Tourette's, what is the message that you would want to share about yourself or the condition in general? Is there anything that comes to mind that makes you think, ***People don't understand my experience as a Touretter and I want them to know what it is like to live with this.*** Is there anything that jumps out at you like that?

Jacob Weiss: I wish people understood that Tourette's doesn't have to be as disruptive as we make it. On the outside, someone might be making a weird facial grimace or contorting their body, but their mind is still functioning like a normal person. We are smart enough to understand what is going on. Our minds can still process thoughts and words, even when our body is making other movements or sounds. So, while it might be hard to completely ignore our tics, you don't have to pause a conversation just because they occur. I can tic and listen at the same time. Maybe my tics will even give you more of a chance to talk, which could be beneficial.

Jason Michaels: Do you feel like most people see you differently than the average person?

Jacob Weiss: I think a lot of times people think that our whole life is lived completely differently, or that we process information in some specialized manner. While some of that might be true, people are still people. We have to go about our lives no matter what condition we were given. Everyone has certain things they must adapt to, even if it's as simple as a left-handed person who gets pencil smudges on their hand while writing. My hope is that people can be more patient, which in turn will make it easier when someone is ticcing. Tics may look strange, but they have nothing to do with someone's ability to understand you or a situation.

Jason Michaels: On the other hand, I believe those of us who live with Tourette's ultimately develop superpowers. You could call these superpowers a trait, gift, or blessing. However you refer to them, tics force you to cultivate certain superpowers, whether it's being hyper-observant, or empathetic, or something else entirely. I, personally, am not sure I would be as empathetic as I am today if I didn't have Tourette's and this life experience.

Do you possess any superpowers that make you think, ***Tourette syndrome has certainly challenged me at times, but it also helped me to develop this trait I love.***

Jacob Weiss: Both the physical and mental parts of Tourette's touches every part of my life. While it is sometimes hard to tell if a trait is Tourette's or OCD, as they blend together, both of those conditions influence the way I generate ideas for research or performances.

The same pathway that breeds OCD-related thoughts is also where creative ideas and connections pop into my head. They feel very similar in the respect that creativity is about making connections between atypical ideas. Similarly, OCD and Tourette's thoughts, like ***if I step my foot a certain way, it will not rain,*** are generally illogical. Just like creativity, these are random connections that don't make rational sense.

When it comes to my work, I believe the same qualities that make me a Touretter are also why I am artistically and intellectually innovative. Even if the ideas that come into my head don't rationally connect, they are what makes performance and research fun. It feels like the creative pathway is the same as Tourette's when I make considerations like, ***What if we applied this messaging system in a way that hasn't been used before?*** Those connections between disparate ideas and neuro pathways through which they arise are very much the same.

Jason Michaels: That's brilliant that your ability to flip things on their head in the arts is the same gene that gives you Tourette's tics. I would imagine making that connection helps you accept them more. Thank you because I had an "a-ha" moment when you were talking. On that same note, has having Tourette's and dealing with tics made you a stronger, more empowered you?

Jacob Weiss: I definitely think it puts you in the mindset of caring less about what others think, which is critical if you want to create art. In a sense, Tourette's has made me more fearless. You try something, realize it's imperfect, and then work to keep improving it. You have to just keep putting yourself out there. Those elements of the creative process, which is about experimenting, definitely tie into how I deal with Tourette's.

Jason Michaels: How do you feel Tourette's has helped you to understand the world more clearly?

Jacob Weiss: Reflecting on what you said about empathy, I am more attuned to people's struggles thanks to Tourette's. Just like my tics aren't always visible on the surface, I realize other people also go through emotions that might not be apparent. Even if I and another person are dealing with different things, empathy allows me to understand their situation.

I feel like my energy and creativity would not be the same if you took away the Tourette's. Whether it is creative thinking or physical movements, like juggling, hand-eye coordination techniques, or basketball, those are all correlated. Similar to how I believe the pathways are the same for Tourette's and creativity, the ability to move quickly, react, and develop muscle memory also comes from the condition.

Most indicative of Tourette's is the preciseness that is imperative for those activities. For example, when I am teaching someone to juggle, it's not about figuring out the height of a throw. Rather, being a skilled juggler is about feeling the motion and right amount of force to put behind the throw. It's about how you catch the ball without gripping it too tightly. There are a lot of creative acts, like writing and playing music, that take just as much subtlety. It's similar to having a feel of the ball when you play

I haven't really thought about it in this way before, but as we're talking, I've realized that Tourette's is often connected with quickness and agility. However, I think in a lot of ways it's more about having a sense of how subtle your movements can be. My Tourette's tics might tell me to flex my hands in a way that isn't too strong or soft. I have to feel the muscle tension at the exact right amount because that's what my tic needs. The ability to have fine control over my movements, and be able to monitor the strength or pressure to the slightest degree, is connected to Tourette's. It is the same goal as getting my tics just right.

To summarize, a lot of the struggle surrounding tics has to do with perfectionism. If you had to clear your throat and hit the exact right vibration the first time, that is probably a one-off. So, you would have to do it again and again to be satisfied. The same goes for flexing your muscles or whatever it is you're doing. You must do it just right. That detailed attention to precision can also result in you being really gifted at sports or performing, for example.

Jason Michaels: Wow, that's quite an insight. You're really firing on all levels here. I was very embarrassed by my tics even until adulthood. What helped me was learning to normalize Tourette's, so the tics just became a part of who I was. *That's just how it is because this is normal for me.* Can you relate to feeling humiliation around your tics?

Jacob Weiss: Yeah, I definitely could feel embarrassed by it. There may have been some situations where I would try to limit how many times I ticced at first, especially if it was someone who I didn't know. As I became more comfortable with someone, I didn't feel as embarrassed if I did tic. It was just a part of who I was.

The embarrassment mostly came down to my disdain for being the focus of a conversation. I didn't want Tourette's to dominate my interactions with others. In some ways, that is probably why I keep my Tourette's separate from my professional life. Playing By Air is a group act for that very reason. I didn't want the performance to be about my own story. I have been intentional throughout my career to never make my Tourette's the topic of conversation. All my time is willingly focused on the show and the group.

Jason Michaels: I have seen your performances many times and consider them to be world class. They are inspiring and beautiful pieces of physical art. The success you've had with your artistic endeavors makes me wonder if you've ever leaned on Tourette's as a way to encourage someone else.

Jacob Weiss: One of the projects that you and I did together was called Tourette Talent. It was designed to highlight the creative talents of Touretters. I wanted to show that you can be more than just the physical or vocal tics that are associated with Tourette's. Those same movements, or vocals, can help Touretters do amazing physical feats or sing beautifully, for example. That project is one of the ways I've uplifted and encouraged other Touretters.

When Playing By Air is touring, sometimes I'll reach out to a Tourette's group and let them know we're performing. I'll say, "Hey, I'm happy to meet with any of the families in the lobby after." Rather than put a major focus on it, I oftentimes encourage people behind the scenes.

I can remember one international performance where a local mom brought her kid to see the show after reading about it in the newspaper. She brought him in and introduced us. We chatted for a bit after the show, which was really nice. I like to encourage kids and believe it's beneficial for them to see someone with Tourette's in the context of a performance. They might not be as comfortable with public speaking and performing themselves. [For] other Touretters, seeing me in that mode is inspiring, even if it's just from the audience. You don't have to meet someone to motivate them.

My sophomore year in college, they created a new student center with a theater in it. We were like, "Hey, why don't we put on a show?" That year kickstarted my ability to put together shows and perform in them. Yet, from the beginning all the way until the present, I always stuck to physical comedy. In the decade that I have been doing this professionally, I never had the confidence to speak on stage. Even if the performances were high-end and the audiences huge, it was all physical comedy.

I had a turning point where I decided to do more keynotes and public speaking. We are still doing the physical comedy-style performances, but I have enjoyed branching out a bit lately. However, it took a long time to gain my confidence as a professional speaker because I never felt like one. I simply look at it as sharing things I'm excited about or that have worked in my own life.

Jason Michaels: Let's say you are in front of a parent whose child has been diagnosed with Tourette's syndrome. I can only imagine how helpless they feel. ***There's nothing I can do*****,** probably runs through their mind. What do they need to know about how to support their child at that moment?

Jacob Weiss: Patience and healthy communication patterns are critical in this situation. Parents must get to the point where they can trust that their child is being truthful about a tic, rather than using it as an excuse for bad behavior. It's easy to assume the worst as an adult. However, if you develop an open line of communication where a child knows they will be believed, then that is a big deal. It will put their mind at ease that you trust their judgment, even if it doesn't make sense from the outside. So, learn to develop both patience and trust, which can be hard for some people to do. Some things, like Tourette's, are simply out of your control.

People with Tourette's or OCD are always trying to get a certain action right. If someone bumps into them while they are trying to get the tic or OCD compulsion exactly right, then they have to start all over. It can be really, really frustrating for them. Your patience comes in if your child gets upset or lashes out from being interrupted. Realize they aren't doing this for fun. The more patient and purposeful you can be in your conversations, the more supportive you can be. Staying in that mode — as opposed to getting frustrated — is helpful.

Jason Michaels: That's great. I want to flip the script. If you're talking to someone who has just been diagnosed with Tourette Syndrome, what do you say to them? How do they deal with it right now?

Jacob Weiss: [I would say,] "Sometimes it's going to be harder to live with it, and other times it's not going to be quite as problematic. Just be patient with yourself, and take the time you need to process the challenging moments. If you're in a mode where you don't want to be around other people, honor that. Try to navigate how you can carve out that alone time for yourself. Lastly, realize that Tourette's is not your identity. It may be a lot of what you're dealing with, but that's not the entirety of what you can do with your life."

"On a day-to-day basis, you can still find ways to do the things you desire. Sometimes it may include adjusting to the situation by holding your tics in or masking them. Yet that isn't necessarily a bad thing. Find your own balance. Try to also set up your home environment so if you do hold it in, you have a space where you can let it all out later. The more you can be patient with yourself, the easier it is to understand Tourette's is part of who you are but not the entire picture."

Jason Michaels: I believe in dreaming big and working towards accomplishing your goals. Do you also find importance in working towards an ambition, or feel it gives your life some sense of purpose? Personally, having huge dreams has provided a sense of direction so I wasn't just focused on my tics. I would sincerely like to ask, "Should someone with Tourette's be aiming for the stars?"

Jacob Weiss: Oh, I definitely think you should be dreaming big dreams. Plus, as we talked about, you have a superpower. You have these abilities that other people can't tap into in quite the same way, which can be used to achieve those big dreams. Many people with Tourette's are super skilled at hyper-focusing on something. This means you should find activities you enjoy doing and see how far you can take them by tapping into that genuine excitement. The interests I got really into were basketball, juggling, and researching how people communicate online. All those activities involve looking at patterns in different ways: the ball handling that basketball entails; the hand-eye coordination skills necessary for juggling patterns; and the communication patterns that develop within online communities. I would go deep into each of my interests, which led to me professionally pursuing a combination of those three today. Yet, I didn't set out to make a profession out of juggling (which I've been doing since age ten), hand-eye coordination exercises, and community building. I just kept doing more of what I enjoyed, getting really deep into the nuances of it, and tried to do a good job. The more you plug in, the easier it is to set up the foundation to do big things.

Even people who don't have a specific grandiose dream for their future still do major things. There isn't one way to live life. If you get really into the activities you love, what once was a little thing on the side could become a catalyst for something major. It could be the momentum that helps you do things in creative ways when you're older.

Jason Michaels: That's wonderful. Is there anything else that you would like to share? The floor is yours.

Jacob Weiss: I didn't take medicine for Tourette's because, fortunately, mine wasn't so extreme that it was debilitating. I could always still function. Yet some days were harder than others, and I had to make adjustments. The turning point was when I realized the connection between my creativity, academic work, and conditions. Recognizing the superpowers I had developed — thanks to my Tourette's neuropathways — was a big deal.

The typical social structures may not be suited to fully empower and utilize those Tourette superpowers. Therefore, it becomes your responsibility to look for ways outside the norm to really tap into them. That's where I think you'll really find confidence, and your abilities will take off. Lean into your superpower even if it doesn't fit into the typical structure of sitting at a desk all day writing, typing, or doing assignments.

Jason Michaels: That's awesome. Absolutely perfect. I really appreciate your willingness to talk about it and to share your insights.

JASON'S SUMMARY

Jacob's insight into using movement to help manage tics is important to note. He said, "I feel very lucky in respect that juggling — which is in a sense like a moving meditation — helped me manage my condition. By juggling for a few hours outdoors after school, all my energy was able to flow through."

As Tourette's is both a physical movement and a vocal tic, using movement to help deal with the tics makes sense. I find myself constantly moving around with a relatively high amount of energy. I believe that finding some sort of physical outlet for it is a good idea.

Jacob's description of the sensory aspects of living with Tourette's was especially interesting. If you are a parent of a Touretter, it can be frustrating when things that seem small or insignificant, such as shoes not being the right weight, can set someone off. If your loved one does happen to go into a highly emotional state, recall what Jacob said, "The sensory aspects of Tourette's and OCD can blend together because that sensitivity and 'right now' feeling where you must get your energy out is very similar."

He continued, "However, I remember having my first Tourette's tics at age four, five and six years. The first indication of it was how long it would take me to pick out a pair of socks that didn't scratch my feet. I'd have to go through a bunch of pairs to find ones that wouldn't bother me."

In order to gracefully handle these episodes, I would recommend following Jacob's advice derived from how his own parents treated him. Jacob said, "My parents were very understanding and patient. I think that patience is one of the key words there."

How is your patience? Do you exhibit tolerance with yourself or with your loved ones even when it is difficult to do so? If not, I recommend further developing this skill as it will allow you to move through the irritating moments with less suffering.

Yet, how do Touretters find healthy ways to cope with their tics? As a creative person, I would lean into Jacob's advice, which is to let go of others' opinions and channel all your energy into artistic hobbies.

Jacob response was, "I definitely think it puts you in the mindset of caring less about what others think, which is critical if you want to create art. In a sense, Tourette's has made me more fearless. You try something, realize it's imperfect, and then work to keep improving it. You have to just keep putting yourself out there. Those elements of the creative process, which is about experimenting, definitely tie into how I deal with Tourette's."

His advice was particularly helpful since many Touretters often go into artistic fields because those fields provide a positive way to channel their energy. As Jacob explained, the same resilience that artists must cultivate is also applicable to Tourette's.

As we grow up, people may begin to try constraining us to fit certain societal expectations. They may want us to acclimate to the often-times confining way they believe life should be lived. But here's the simple truth: you can do whatever you like. You get to decide the course you take, the passions and profession you pursue, and the direction you take yourself in. Remember when Jacob said the following: "The typical social structures may not be suited to fully empower and utilize those Tourette superpowers. Therefore, it becomes your responsibility to look for ways outside the norm to really tap into them. That's where I think you'll really find confidence, and your abilities will take off. Lean into your superpower even if it doesn't fit into the typical structure of sitting at a desk all day writing, typing, or doing assignments."

It's not always easy to blaze your own trail in life, but the experience will always be incredibly fulfilling. Going against the grain might be exactly what you need to become the person you were fully designed to be. As a professional magician and keynote speaker, I certainly took the path less traveled, and that has made all the difference*.

---

*This famous closing line from Robert Frost's 1915 poem "The Road Not Taken" signifies the profound impact of choosing a less conventional path in life. It highlights the importance of individual choice, independence, and courage, suggesting that unconventional decisions, despite potential difficulties, lead to significant, life-altering outcomes.

To watch the video of the full interview with Jacob Weiss, access additional tools to help you live and thrive with Tourette Syndrome, and connect with the Tourette Warrior community, please visit TouretteWarrior.com.

In the next chapter, my interview with David Shenton, the legendary musician and composer shares some of his coping mechanisms when dealing with tics. He also discusses how he built up his confidence, which has been critical to his success, and developed the superpowers of sensitivity, empathy, and active listening.

CHAPTER 7

DAVID SHENTON

WORLD-CLASS MUSICIAN AND COMPOSER

David Shenton is an accomplished British pianist, violinist, composer, and arranger who is now based in New York City. He has collaborated with renowned artists across multiple genres, including Tony Bennett, Vanessa Williams, Renée Fleming, and Alan Menken. His sonic versatility has provided opportunities to perform at prestigious venues worldwide. Most notably this includes Carnegie Hall, where he made his debut in 2014, conducting his own orchestra and big band. He has also performed at Lincoln Center and that respective venue's Rubenstein Atrium, showcasing his talent in both jazz and classical music. As a violinist, he shined on his own as a soloist playing with leading orchestras. His work as an arranger and orchestrator has been featured in Hollywood films, Broadway plays, and London's esteemed West End, including The Snowman, which has been running at the TKTK theatre since 1998.

In addition to his performance career, Shenton is a prolific composer, having written a symphony, concertos, musicals, and film scores. He co-founded the classical crossover act Empire Trio with his wife, soprano Erin Shields, and baritone Adam Cannedy, and has created numerous shows, including a Lincoln Center-commissioned production on Italian popular music. His collaborations with lyricist Martin Charnin resulted in over a dozen musical revues featuring Broadway talent. As an educator, he has served on the faculties of NYU, The New School, and The Lee Strasberg Theatre & Film Institute, and he continues to mentor the next generation of musicians as Music Director at

Grace Church School. A graduate of the Royal College of Music in London, Shenton remains a sought-after talent and composer in both classical and contemporary circles in the states and abroad.

Jason Michaels: David, you are this incredibly prolific musician. You play multiple instruments, are a composer, an arranger, and a producer. You live in New York City where you've collaborated with all sorts of musicians and celebrities there and beyond. You have highlights that are just incredibly impressive, so I want to hear about that. Not being a musician myself, I probably don't understand the caliber of your accomplishments, but I know we can all learn from your life experience. Please share a little bit about yourself.

David Shenton: I started playing the violin at the age of seven. I was literally just given a violin in school one day and told, "This is the way that it's going to be. We need three kids in every classroom to play an instrument." Mine was the violin. It was determined the first time we did a musical experiment that I had perfect pitch. Of course, they wanted me to carry on, and I took the violin home that day. Prior to this, I didn't even know what a violin looked like. It was just a big block of wood that I really loved playing. Ironically, I was really into rock 'n' roll at the time, which my twin brother and two sisters also listened to, until my parents introduced me to classical music. That genre changed my life.

From that point on, since I was a fairly introverted kid, I would read musical scores instead of story books. That gave me a greater understanding of the language of music, which allowed me to excel faster at my craft later in life. I could essentially pick up any score, read it, and literally hear the notes coming off the page. While that's nothing special to most conductors and composers, at that age my gifts were considered exceptional.

Jason Michaels: Yet you had an injury that caused you to pivot early on in your career. How did you handle that?

David Shenton: At one point my parents said, "You should probably play the piano." I started learning the piano at just shy of age thirteen and studied at the Royal College of Music in London some years later.

I excelled in both instruments and started getting calls to play with orchestras and all sorts of wonderful ensembles. As a violinist, I played a lot of concertos with orchestras. The last concert I ever did was to play the Mendelssohn Violin Concerto with a big symphony orchestra, which was a career highlight. However, my violin career was ultimately cut short because of a finger injury. The piano, I could continue with; and as a result, I ended up playing in fancy hotels and bars in London.

One day this guy approached me and said, "Do you write music?" I said yes because I'd also written music from the age of nine. That meeting led to me writing my first "Broadway show," which I put in quotes because it didn't go to Broadway, but rather off-off-Broadway, and then subsequently off-Broadway. That turning point was basically the impetus for me wanting to move to New York.

Jason Michaels: Did you immediately start getting paid for gigs in NYC?

David Shenton: When I first moved to New York, I started playing in a nightclub where someone approached me one evening and asked, "Can you do a gig with me in Staten Island?" Turns out we were opening for Tony Bennett, and that was literally a couple of years after I moved to the States. It's one of those situations where I thought, ***Wow, this is the country of dreams***. While my career was going fine in England, I always wanted something more. Then, within a couple of years, I'd already done that huge, high-stakes gig. Some of my other highlights are working with legends like Vanessa Williams one-on-one and over 300 Broadway singers. I also arranged music for Andre Previn* and Michael Feinstein's* album.

I've worked with Pinchas Zukerman*, who's a great violinist, and Igor Oistrakh*. Renee Fleming* has sung my works; and then, Stephen Schwartz*, Alan Menken*, a lot of these big Broadway composers, all of whom I've worked with directly or indirectly. I've worked with Paul McCartney.

I also played with a massive ensemble in London, the John Wilson Orchestra, of which I was a founding member. In my opinion, it is one of the greatest symphony orchestras, and I was able to do a lot of fun performances with them. Yet, while the name-recognition and accomplishments might be impressive, I am most proud of the adversity I've overcome. Simply getting on stage every day, even though I do it a couple hundred times a year, is a tremendous feat for me. Also, receiving recognition for my compositions, which I've been writing since age nine, has been especially meaningful.

During the pandemic I wrote two full-length operas, which have subsequently been produced multiple times. The fact that I am finally getting recognition for my own voice in the music world is probably my proudest achievement so far.

Every day I'm getting more calls. Empire Trio has already had close to thirty-five shows this year, and I'm going on tour again next week. Then, I have another twenty shows. We're incredibly busy, and I'm incredibly grateful for that. I could name-drop all the celebrities I've played for in private party situations, or say the household names I've shared piano benches with, but that isn't necessarily the highlight for me. Most impressive is the fact that I have a voice in the music world and had to overcome a tremendous amount of adversity to earn that recognition.

It's sort of like the difference between opera and musicals, of which I've written eleven. While I have only written two operas, they are the compositions I'm most proud of because the craftsmanship must be at a much higher level. It's just a more sophisticated art form. I don't mean to bastardize Broadway, but it's the equivalent of eating a McDonald's hamburger — versus opera, which is like savoring a delicate filet mignon in a fancy steakhouse. From orchestrating Broadway shows before, I know that their arrangements aren't nearly as complex as the classical music world. That intellectual hierarchy is why I am proudest of the classical accomplishments.

Jason Michaels: It sounds like you're operating at the most elite level in your field. Yet, on the other hand, it is easy to worry as a young person with Tourette Syndrome that the tics will limit you. While you have clearly pushed through those potential roadblocks, do you ever feel anxiety when performing on stage? How does that affect you?

David Shenton: I mean, what some people could call anxiety, I see to a certain degree as acknowledging that I have no control over my body. When I'm backstage, as my wife will tell you, I'm all over the place. My body goes into overdrive because I know in a couple of minutes, or even seconds, I'll walk onto a stage with nothing to hide behind. It will just be me, a piano, and a couple of microphones with 1,000 people staring right at me. That is the worst. Ironically, as much as I love to perform, when I go to a restaurant, I ask for the corner table. In the movie theater, I sit in the back seat. I will do anything to make sure I receive zero attention.

Jason Michaels: That reminds me of actors who say they are super shy but are dynamic on the stage or screen.

David Shenton: If I go and see a concert or a Broadway show, I want to get a good seat naturally. Then, I will kind of slouch in my chair, even if the person in front obscures my view. I've got this defense mechanism about certain situations.

Fortunately, my tics haven't severely impacted my career. I remember a pianist who was also at the Royal College of Music a few years before me. Their career literally ended because they couldn't stop keybedding, which means they would push into it with too much force while playing a concerto. This person unfortunately couldn't play because of how badly their hands spasmed.

The lack of physical control you have over Tourette's is the most infuriating thing about it. Even if it appears like I'm performing incredibly well on stage, there is always an OCD moment. It might be something small, like my finger has to touch the middle C at a certain point. Still, that desire overtakes everything.

Trying to really get into the performance and have both channels of my brain to deal with can be a challenge. I always say that my mind is divided into two: the left side of the brain, which is logical, and the right side of the brain for the artistic endeavors. One side is working on the performance, and the other is trying to figure out how to deal with my tics. When both channels are aligned and working towards the music, I can get completely lost in it. My tics go away and I'm free. After those glorious moments, I always walk offstage thinking, ***Wow, I did it again,*** because it's so unexpected. At this point, I've clocked in 4,500 performances, which means the same number of experiences where everything coalesces. Yet I still don't expect it. I can't remember a time when I've walked onstage and not felt some sort of anxiety. I often wonder, ***What are people going to say?***

Jason Michaels: We have all struggled with caring what others think, but how do you put this aside in order to deliver?

David Shenton: Fortunately, I've gotten to the point where I really don't care what people say, even if it's negative, or they are offensive. I've kind of come to terms with the fact that I have no control over that. Yet the battle I am always facing is knowing my potential when I'm fully relaxed and understanding the chances of that happening are 50/50. I've got certain mechanisms. There are certain technical things I can do on the piano which I've practiced 10,000 times that sound incredibly impressive. If I get a hint that some kind of neurological symptom is about to expose itself, I'll just do something on the piano to elicit a burst of appreciation from the audience. It takes the concentration off me for a second so I can have that time to tic. Thanks to the stress, I've had to adapt how I perform on a daily basis.

Jason Michaels: That's fascinating and mirrors many of the other conversations I've had where Touretters explain ways they've learned to deflect, distract, or adapt. They've developed their own little tricks based on their personal experiences to fulfill the Tourette tics.

Switching gears a bit, seeing as you are originally from the United Kingdom, is there a palpable difference in the way you are treated there versus the States? How do you feel society handles your Tourette's back home versus in the United States?

David Shenton: Honestly, when I moved to the States, while I missed my family like crazy, I knew that I wanted to stay here because of the high tolerance level. The openness of American society, particularly to conditions like Tourette's, has really inspired me. In England, the stiff-upper-lip syndrome is for real. People just don't talk about their problems of any sort quite as much. I was subjected to a lot of bullying, taunting, and gossiping even by my best friends, peers, and colleagues. My closest friend I once overheard talking about me in the back seat of a taxi as I sat in front chatting with the driver. He wasn't overly cautious about it, which was perhaps the most devastating thing of all. I realized at that moment that I couldn't even talk to my closest friend about my condition. My family would also generally brush it under the carpet, too.

Jason Michaels: How do you find the treatment of people who have Tourette's differs in America?

David Shenton: That's just basically the way it is in England. People don't really wear their hearts on their sleeves as much as they do in America. I found that people don't know how to deal with it. Awkward questions are particularly taboo in England; whereas in the States, I found that people would just come up and ask, "Hey, what's with the tics?" Americans, as is their reputation, are just more direct. I appreciate this because it forces me to open up instead of going back into my shell, which is something I did quite a lot of in England.

Jason Michaels: What was one of the most upsetting situations you ever experienced in regard to Tourette's being made fun of or ignored?

David Shenton: I taught for a few years at a very prestigious boys' choir school in New York where, ironically, the choir master was English. One of my violin students, who is still my mentee to this day, had severe tics which no one at the school knew how to handle. So, I wrote to the headmaster and said that I would be willing to step up to the plate and help. After he shot my idea down, I found out not too long after that the choir master had been mimicking this poor student's tics. I ended up leaving that job because I couldn't be in an environment where abuse and bullying were condoned.

Unfortunately, that same choir master passed away at the age of fifty-six from a heart attack, which was tragic because of how talented he was. However, I will never understand why someone of that age and level of respect in the music industry could behave with such cruelty. He found it necessary, or even funny, to mimic someone who's obviously overcoming major personal challenges. Going full circle, the way some English people deal with uncomfortable situations just wasn't right for me. Where I grew up in the north, in a small mining town, they would either ignore my condition or make fun of it. There was no in-between.

Jason Michaels: Has an audience member ever confronted you about your tics?

David Shenton: I can't really comment on the difference between interacting with American and English audiences because it never happens in England. When I perform there, you don't speak to the audience after the show. That's one thing we always do in the States because straight after the show you go out into the lobby to sell your CDs and merchandise. In England, especially when you play classical music, you go on stage, do a show, and then leave. My current shows are much more interactive, which creates an even deeper relationship with the audience. However, throughout the hundreds of performances we've done in America, I can't remember anyone ever approaching me about my tics. I feel much more comfortable here with the whole social mentality, particularly when it relates to Tourette's.

Jason Michaels: Whether it has to do with education or awareness, I've heard other stories about similar intolerance which were upsetting. Let's dive into your childhood for a bit. Did tics suddenly arise out of nowhere, or do they go back as far as you can remember?

David Shenton: It's been happening as long as I can remember. Oddly enough, I have an identical twin brother who also had basic tics growing up. For some reason, they completely left him.

Jason Michaels: Wow.

David Shenton: His variation was never as bad as mine and was most restricted to less severe behaviors like rapid eye blinking. Maybe it was because he was more confident than I was. He did karate and was tough, which might have impacted his tics' ability to stick around. The earliest memory I have surrounding my own tics was in kindergarten. These two girls in my class came over, stopped, and stared at me for a while. Then they started whispering in each other's ears saying, "Watch, he's going to do it!" Then they would start laughing at how I was uncontrollably shaking my head. While I knew something was wrong, I wasn't sure what caused it. From there, I went to see my parents who already knew what was going on. I love my parents deeply, but for some reason they pretended like they didn't notice my tics.

They always thought my Tourette's would go away eventually; but for a kid growing up, it's a very tough condition to have. On a more positive note, I remember the first time I saw the piano in the gymnasium at my kindergarten. The teacher used to play a hymn before assembly every morning. I just remember it looking like a big box in the corner. Then, fast-forward two years later, I started playing the violin, which became like my best friend. I had to practice, an action that kept my mind occupied and off the tics. That was probably the reason I liked it so much. Sadly, the bullying I endured from age five through the end of high school made me incredibly introverted. It was a very difficult time, and I hid away with my violin.

Jason Michaels: I'm so sorry you had to go through that.

David Shenton: I spent a lot of time in the library just reading music scores and that kind of thing. Again, I wish my parents had handled it differently as I believe that would have given me more confidence. However, in the end I choose not to let their choices bother me. I am who I am because of Tourette's, which is an incredibly sensitive person who is more aware than most of everything around me. Most fortunately, I can tell in an instant if someone has Tourette's and is willing to talk about it. I want to help people who are open to my guidance, which is why I was a mentor for the Tourette Syndrome Association for a few years.

Jason Michaels: When you are playing and practicing the violin, do you feel that your tics are suppressed because of the sole focus on what you're doing at that moment? Or do you remember still having tics while you played?

David Shenton: I'd say probably 60/40. Sixty percent of the time I was completely engrossed in playing the violin, which meant that both channels of my mind were focused on the instrument. Playing an instrument involves repetition. While in college, I was expected to practice the violin for six to eight hours a day and also spend two to three hours on the piano. That's a lot of hours. What helped me a lot was watching a movie while I practiced. I would sit down, open a study book, and then go through the motions with my fingers. Completely concentrating on both the movie and violin meant that both parts of my mind were fully occupied. The second the movie switched off, the tics would start up because that channel of my mind opened back up. Sixty percent of the time I wouldn't have tics, and forty percent of the time my mind would wander off probably due to my ADHD and OCD. The second my mind wanders off a subject, it's almost like a switch turns on the tics. Knowing that they will keep coming back, I try to keep my mind as fully occupied as I can throughout the day through cerebral exercises, crosswords, or Wordle. I do whatever it takes to help me concentrate on a specific task. That feeling of complete concentration is what I try to take and attribute to the process of music making.

I am not sure what it is like for you, but once in a blue moon, the tics get bad. For me, it goes in cycles where they go away and then come back again. It's almost like a season, and when I am in the depths of despair, I can't really do anything physically. It's incredibly infuriating so I just try to relax, have a cup of tea, and do some breathing exercises. When it's the opposite and the tics go away, I am most productive and can truly concentrate on writing and arranging music. My life is basically scheduled around my body acting however it wants to.

Jason Michaels: Knowing how difficult some of your life has been, do you recall a time when someone acted as a champion for you? During those tough times, did anyone stand up for you or even just go, "Hey, it's going to be okay. Just keep plugging along."

David Shenton: That's a tricky question. As far as my career goes, my mom and dad for sure; but regarding Tourette's, unfortunately no.

Jason Michaels: So you had to learn how to be resilient on your own, didn't you?

David Shenton: Actually, I can think of one person in England [who encouraged me]. To set the scene, I played in this fancy restaurant and bar in London called Le Caprice, where every night someone famous would walk through the door. Princess Diana, Elton John, Bill Clinton, Arnold Schwarzenegger, you name it. I could write a whole book about what celebrities did and shouldn't have been doing because the number I met there was just off the charts. I saw people lining up spliffs, getting drunk and falling off tables, and even Royal Family members trying to order a bottle of whiskey from the bar. It was hilarious.

The gentleman I mentioned, Alan Taylor, looked like a grand wizard. He wore fancy clothes and had long white hair with a balding crown up top. Turns out he was an entrepreneur who started the phenomenon of text messaging. This man, with many business interests, was also a gazillionaire. Every night, he'd come in and stick fifty to upwards of three hundred pounds in cash in my top jacket pocket as he left. He was incredibly generous and even took me and three colleagues to Gordon Ramsay's restaurant in Claridge's one night. Ramsay had just won his third Michelin star and was there that evening. He also used to come into Le Caprice as a patron all the time.

That evening, I had an incredible tic attack while everyone in the restaurant looked on. Even Gordon Ramsay was staring at me and trying to figure out what to do because the whole situation was such a distraction. Fortunately, we were allowed to stay, which was incredibly kind because I can't imagine what the whole scene looked like. My head was just throwing back uncontrollably. The next day Alan called me and said, "We need to talk. What's wrong with you?" I told him about my Tourette's after which he said, "You should probably see a therapist." From there on out, he wrote me regular emails of encouragement and even produced and financed an entire recording project of mine. He gave me quite a bit of money for that.

His friendship made me realize that Tourette's was nothing to be ashamed of. It doesn't matter what you've got if you have the talent that allows you to proceed with your ambitions. I am incredibly grateful for him.

Shortly after that I moved to the States and met Erin, my wife, who immediately said, "Okay, we've got to talk about this, whatever it is." That's when I started talking about it. While I don't mean to sound melodramatic, Erin saved my life in some ways by giving me the courage to open up about my condition. She always championed me by saying, "Who cares what people think? It's their problem." She would constantly remind me to go after my goals and that I had the talent to do it. Her belief is why I kept going and pushing forward.

Those are the main people, besides my parents, who were the most supportive in terms of my career. However, when it came to Tourette's — as the English way goes — my parents, unfortunately, didn't want to acknowledge what was happening. So, thank you to Alan Taylor, who gave me the confidence to write and record a show and then move to New York, where I met Erin. My wife, I would say, has been my greatest champion.

Jason Michaels: Would I be right in saying that the tough, British stiff-upper-lip mentality helped you accept Tourette's in your formative years, but the massive turning point was, ironically, being able to open up about it?

David Shenton: Yeah, but it wasn't overnight. It took a few years for me to gain the confidence to open up. Now I don't mind opening up about Tourette's at all; however, had you asked me to do this interview twenty years ago, I probably would have said no. Today, I care and then kind of don't. I remember going to my first Tourette Association Conference where a well-known jazz pianist spoke and absolutely captured how I feel. He said, "It's not something I am ashamed of, but I certainly don't advertise it. If people want to know more, they can ask." Similarly, if people look at me funny, I try to put it into perspective. There's a lot more important things in this world to worry about than a stranger's opinion. So, getting back to your original question, I would say the way you described my turning point is accurate.

Jason Michaels: Can you think of a particular situation where a friend severely misunderstood the nature of your Tourette's?

David Shenton: In England, I had two best friends: the one from home who hurt my feelings when he spoke about my condition in a derogatory manner; and my best friend from the Royal College who was morbidly obese. The latter used to call me "Twitch," which was very upsetting. Finally, one day I said, "Please stop calling me that," to which he responded, "What's wrong, Twitch?" I couldn't take it anymore and said, "Okay, I'm going to call you Fatso then." He pushed me and explained that he couldn't help his weight, which clearly wasn't true. I was like, "Well then, you really don't understand Tourette's because it literally is uncontrollable versus your weight, which is." Since then, subsequently, he has undergone surgery to remove the excess weight which proves his situation was fixable. It is why education around Tourette's is so important because, unfortunately, some people assume you are just ticking for fun.

Jason Michaels: You're so right. While there is a greater awareness surrounding Tourette's today, there is still a level of education that society lacks. Speaking to the positive, would you say that Tourette's has ever benefitted a part of your life. Are there any elements you can look at and say, "Thanks to Tourette's, I am better at this."

David Shenton: I think in terms of my musical "abilities," those are definitely all Tourette's related. Tourette's often comes hand in hand with OCD, which makes you inclined to do something repeatedly to make it perfect. That's how I got in my 10,000 hours because when they say you need to do that to be good at the violin, they're not joking. You must play a piece hundreds of times before you can present it to the public. To be able to apply my OCD to the mentality of practicing really helped my abilities. On another note, being what I would call an empath or highly empathetic is also a positive attribute related to Tourette's. I am so aware of other people's emotions because of my incredible self-awareness. While I sometimes feel that I am overly sensitive and care way too much, it is also why I am a very good listener. I never want to give someone a negative impression. Thanks to the attention I've received over the years when people stared at me while I ticked, I have the same level of empathy for others' problems. It has helped me to be there for friends, and sometimes even strangers, maybe to a fault. My wife always says, "You're too nice to everybody," which probably stems from my childhood.

The other thing that I can think of is how my mind, thanks to OCD, never really switches off. I spoke to a Broadway composer, David Shire, about it once. We chatted about how if you have a music-related problem, somewhere the back of your mind is always trying to work it out. Let's say it's an orchestration, a fugue or song you're writing, or a melody you can't put your finger on. You put it away to the back of your mind where it continues germinating. Suddenly, the answer pops into the front of your head! I'm consciously aware of that process and believe music is going through my mind every minute of the day, which sometimes drives me crazy. However, it is related to my neurological symptoms and is inevitably a good thing. I am always in that mode of trying to figure out musical conundrums.

For example, last week I was working with Jane Monheit, a well-known jazz singer. I was very nervous about working together because she is a legend. I, on the other hand, am not really a jazz pianist because I am a classically trained musician, even though I've been playing the genre for twenty-five years. For the few weeks leading up to our performance, I kept going over the songs in my head over and over. I've managed to manifest that the part of my brain where tics comes from can also produce a repetitive sort of thought process. The reason the concert was so successful is because I literally ran through each song hundreds of times in my brain prior to performing. By the time we arrived onstage, I knew each song by memory and could also anticipate what she was going to do. I just knew what would sound good.

In terms of musical ability, this quirk has helped a lot. I always say it would be nice to live without it, but I think if I ever did get cured, I would eliminate an essential part of my personality. Instead, I have chosen to be happy with who I truly am. I want to let other people who are suffering know that they should also be at peace with themselves because everyone is perfect in their own way.

JASON'S SUMMARY

I find it interesting how different Touretters use different coping mechanisms. Personally, David's approach feels like the one that I often take. These comments of his struck a chord with me: "Ironically, as much as I love to perform, when I go to a restaurant, I ask for the corner table. In the movie theater, I sit in the back seat. I will do anything to make sure I receive zero attention."

Similarly, I have found that sometimes it is just too exhausting to educate the world about Tourette's. That is a perfectly acceptable reason to try and blend in with your surroundings and to seek out public areas that may be a little more private.

Several of the interviews that I've done have referenced CBIT* or have described coping strategies that are similar to what this methodology teaches us. David's description of coping with tics while playing the piano is particularly notable. He said, "I've got certain mechanisms. There are certain technical things I can do on the piano which I've practiced 10,000 times that sound incredibly impressive. If I get a hint that some kind of neurological symptom is about to expose itself, I'll just do something on the piano to elicit a burst of appreciation from the audience. It takes the concentration off me for a second so I can have that time to tic. Thanks to the stress, I've had to adapt how I perform on a daily basis." This comment also makes me think of how magicians use misdirection to focus your attention on what they want you to see, instead of where the sleight-of-hand may be occurring.

I often encourage people to open up willingly about their struggles. Communicating your struggles is a very therapeutic thing to do, and it helps normalize living with Tourette Syndrome. The simple truth is that other people won't know what it's like to live with tics unless they have a similar condition. Explaining it to them helps them empathize with you. Unfortunately, people will still be people, and sometimes your closest friends and family will let you down.

The following comment about David's inner circle was disappointing to hear. "My closest friend I once overheard talking about me in the back seat of a taxi as I sat in front chatting with the driver. He wasn't overly cautious about it, which was perhaps the most devastating thing of all. I realized at that moment that I couldn't even talk to my closest friend about my condition. My family would also generally brush it under the carpet, too."

I can feel the pain that this admission must stir up in David, and I am thankful that he chose to share it with us. His example is powerful because it shows us that we are not alone when we feel hurt, disappointed, or let down. David's friend and some of his family members did not acknowledge his struggles in the way that David would have preferred; yet by him sharing this grievance, I hope it makes others living with Tourette's feel less alone. David is just like us, which means we are never really alone in our journey.

In fact, I believe these next comments from David are an excellent example of how he redirected his difficulties to help others. He said, "Sadly, the bullying I endured from age five through the end of high school made me incredibly introverted. It was a very difficult time, and I hid away with my violin."

He continued, "I spent a lot of time in the library just reading music scores and that kind of thing. Again, I wish my parents had handled it differently as I believe that would have given me more confidence. However, in the end I choose not to let their choices bother me. I am who I am because of Tourette's, which is an incredibly sensitive person who is more aware than most of everything around me. Most fortunately, I can tell in an instant if someone has Tourette's and is willing to talk about it."

What an incredible example that David sets for us. Empathy and compassion are both foundational traits in the development of resilience. It appears David learned these traits by actively living his life. He has stepped into the fire time and again, which has made him sensitive to the issues of others in an almost superhuman way. People who meet David are fortunate to cross such a good listener's path when dealing with their own struggles.

I am so pleased that Alan Taylor, a generous patron of the arts and wealthy businessman, has been a part of David's life. It is obvious from David's comments that Alan, and later his wife Erin, have made such a major impact in his life. Knowing that others are willing to stand up for you as champions can be life-changing. It makes you feel like you don't have to hold up the whole machine on your own. David said, "His (Alan Taylor's) friendship made me realize that Tourette's was nothing to be ashamed of. It doesn't matter what you've got if you have the talent that allows you to proceed with your ambitions. I am incredibly grateful for him."

At one point in the interview I asked the following, "Would I be right in saying that the tough, British stiff-upper-lip mentality helped you accept Tourette's in your formative years, but the massive turning point was, ironically, being able to open up about it?"

David response was about as honest as it gets, "Yeah, but it wasn't overnight. It took a few years for me to gain the confidence to open up." I think that is important to remember because we often want immediate results. The journey of life is one that happens over time. Sometimes that means that it takes much longer than we think it should to get to the place where we want to be. Keep that in mind the next time you get frustrated with something going on in your life whether it involves accepting tics or not.

It is important to note that David and I grew up during a different generation than now. The education for those of us with Tourette's was not what it is today. With that said, however, it is important to keep in mind his comment, "It is why education around Tourette's is so important because, unfortunately, some people assume you are just ticking for fun."

Sadly, it falls to those of us with Tourette's, and the people who love us, to educate others about our condition. Just for the record, that doesn't mean that it will be easy. Everyone has a very limited perspective based on their specific life experience. When and if you ever come across someone who doesn't acknowledge your struggle, ask yourself this question, "I wonder what this person is going through?" I promise you they are struggling with something that probably has nothing to do with you. This might be infringing upon their ability to empathize with your situation.

I believe that this comment from David, meant to speak to the positive traits of Tourette's, backs up that claim: "On another note, being what I would call an empath or highly empathetic is also a positive attribute related to Tourette's. I am so aware of other people's emotions because of my incredible self-awareness. While I sometimes feel that I am overly sensitive and care way too much, it is also why I am a very good listener. I never want to give someone a negative impression. Thanks to the attention I've received over the years when people stared at me while I ticked, I have the same level of empathy for others' problems. It has helped me to be there for friends, and sometimes even strangers."

There are all kinds of gifts that will naturally be bestowed upon us Touretters. Empathy, sympathy, and compassion are ones that make the world a much better place. Please keep this in mind on the tough days. Thanks to your own trials, you might just become the best friend someone else needs to get through theirs.

These final comments from David pretty much sum up the message of this book, which is that Tourette's oftentimes makes us into real-life superheroes: "I always say it would be nice to live without it, but I think if I ever did get cured, I would eliminate an essential part of my personality. Instead, I have chosen to be happy with who I truly am. I want to let other people who are suffering know that they should also be at peace with themselves because everyone is perfect in their own way."

---

*Andre Previn (April 6, 1929-February 28, 2019) was a German and American conductor, composer, and pianist. (Wikipedia)

*Michael Feinstein is an American singer, pianist, and music revivalist. He is an archivist and interpreter for the repertoire known as the Great American Songbook. (Wikipedia)

*Pinchas Zukerman is an Israeli-American violinist, violist and conductor. (Wikipedia)

*Igor Oistrakh (April 1931-August 14, 2021) was a Soviet and Russian violinist. He was described by Encyclopedia Britannica as "noted for his lean, modernist interpretations". (Wikipedia)

*Renee Fleming is an American soprano and actress, known for performances in opera, concerts, recordings, theater, film, and at major public occasions. (Wikipedia)

*Stephen Schwartz is an American musical theatre composer and lyricist. In a career spanning over five decades, Schwartz has written hit musicals including Godspell, Pippin, and Wicked. (Wikipedia)

*Alan Menken is an American composer and conductor. Over his career he has received numerous accolades including winning eight Academy Awards, a Tony Award, eleven Grammy Awards, seven Golden Globe Awards, and a Daytime Emmy Award. He is one of twenty-two recipients to have won the competitive EGOT. (Wikipedia)

*Comprehensive Behavioral Intervention for Tics (CBIT) is a structured, non-drug therapy for reducing tic severity in children and adults with Tourette Syndrome and chronic tic disorders. It involves habit reversal training (identifying urges and using competing responses), relaxation techniques, and environmental adjustments to manage tics.

To watch the video of the full interview with David Shenton, access additional tools to help you live and thrive with Tourette Syndrome, and connect with the Tourette Warrior community, please visit TouretteWarrior.com.

In the next chapter, the interview with Dave Pittman, the singer and recording artist gets very raw, honest, and open. He discusses a suicide attempt and how his faith brought him closer to his Creator during this challenging time. Religion also gave him purpose. He also discusses the incredible difference between "accepting" and "embracing" living with Tourette Syndrome, which can be a true game-changer.

CHAPTER 8

DAVE PITTMAN

SINGER AND RECORDING ARTIST

Dave Pittman is a gifted singer-songwriter with a world-class voice and an inspiring story of resilience. Diagnosed with Tourette Syndrome at a young age, he faced relentless bullying that led him to a dark moment at just ten years old. However, his journey didn't end there. Instead, he emerged stronger, using his experiences to uplift others through music and storytelling. As a former American Idol contestant, Dave has captivated audiences nationwide, turning his trials into triumphs. Today, he continues to be a beacon of hope, using his voice to inspire and encourage others.

Jason Michaels: Where did you grow up, and what was that like for you?

Dave Pittman: My tics started showing up when I was seven years old. I think one of my first tics was blinking my eyes and twitching my nose. My parents noticed and thought it was a bad habit at first. They were trying to figure out what their seven-year-old son was doing since my behavior seemed abnormal.

Sometimes they would discipline me because they were trying to help me break a habit. Let me preface this by saying, "I have great parents. They were just trying to do the best thing they could to help me in those early years."

From ages seven to nine was when I was diagnosed. It was a long process of trying to figure out what was causing the tics.

I saw doctor after doctor: neurologists, psychologists, all types. A neurologist in Little Rock, Arkansas, at Little Rock Baptist Children's Hospital finally diagnosed me with Tourette's. I think for me, knowing is half the battle. At first, you're thinking, ***What is this?*** Then you find out exactly what your diagnosis is. A huge weight is lifted, until you move on to ask, ***How do I manage it?*** **Then, *What do I do to treat it? If there is such a thing.***

So, that was extremely difficult. It was good news, but scary news because I didn't know how we were going to move forward.

Jason Michaels: How did this huge diagnosis hanging over your head affect your ability to feel normal?

Dave Pittman: Honestly, my childhood was difficult, especially after the diagnosis which happened at age nine when I was in the fourth grade. My tics made me a target for bullying. A lot of my peers would make fun of me, calling me names like "Spaz Boy" and things like that. They would mimic me by copying some of the things I did like shaking my head. It hurt deeply.

Jason Michaels: Of course, brutal.

Dave Pittman: Yeah. Plus, I never really opened up to my parents about how negatively it affected me.

Jason Michaels: The bullying?

Dave Pittman: The bullying and how I was dealing with it overall. I couldn't understand why this was happening to me. I felt targeted by my peers, but also from God.

I was like, "Well, God, why would you allow me to have this thing? Why not my sister or brother? Why not them? Why me?"

One morning prior to the start of fifth grade, I was sitting at the breakfast table with my parents and siblings. My mom said, "Are you guys ready to go back to school? It starts in the next two weeks."

My mom still remembers the terror that came over my face like, ***There's no way I can go back and face another year of what I already went through.***

In that moment, I was more afraid of living than dying, and I became suicidal. I was ready to take my life. Of course, my mom said, "Well Dave, you have to go back to school. You can't just opt out. You have to go back."

Jason Michaels: And this is at nine years old?

Dave Pittman: Actually, I was ten at this time.

My parents left later that afternoon to run an errand. As soon as they did, I went back to my room and got a piece of paper and a pencil and wrote down, "Mom and Dad, I love you. I'm going to miss you."

I drew a frown face with a tear rolling down. From there, I went to my mom and dad's room, shut and locked the door, and put the note face up. I got my dad's gun, and I was about two seconds from pulling the trigger. I counted one, two, and then I heard the door of our home open. Knowing that mom and dad had come home sooner than I had expected stopped me. I put the note face down and scurried around to get things back in order.

My mom and dad walked down the hallway and knocked on the door because I had locked it. They nervously said, "Dave, what are you doing?" My siblings were in another part of the house, so they didn't know what was going on.

They tried to get into the room after I had just gotten things back in order. So I let them in, and they asked me, "Dave, why were you in here with the door locked?"

I wasn't going to tell them what I had planned. That is until my mom looked around and saw the piece of paper on the floor. Sadly, she turned it over and saw the horror that was written on the other side.

She just lost it and so did I. All those feelings from the prior year came out. So, we had a moment in the middle of their bedroom floor where we prayed together. Finally, to make a long story short, they got me into counseling to help me work through some of my Tourette's related issues.

Jason Michaels: Did your parents make any other changes to improve your situation?

Dave Pittman: Mom and Dad decided to pull me out of public school and homeschool me that next year for the fifth grade. That was a hard year for Mom and me because she had never home-schooled anybody before. I, of course, had never gone through the homeschooling process.

That year, I just remember Mom and Dad drilling into my head, into my heart, the importance of accepting yourself for who you are. As a believer, they showed me that what truly mattered wasn't just who I was in the world — but rather who I was in Jesus Christ. That's my story and the reason behind my relationship with Christ.

Jason Michaels: I love the fact that you have that relationship with Jesus and are completely unafraid to talk about it. That's wonderful.

Dave Pittman: Well, my strength comes from Him. That's ultimately the purpose behind my music. I go and share my story as a way of bringing a bit of hope to the world.

The world's so lost. There's no hope, but rather so much hate and a misunderstanding of identity. Being able to connect with others provided some of my "me" questions with answers. Prior to that, I couldn't understand why God allowed me to have Tourette's.

I remember my mom telling me something profound which was, "Dave, we may not understand why God allowed you to have Tourette's. We don't even really know exactly what it is yet." Then she said, "But you've got a couple of choices. You can be completely miserable — have no joy, peace, or happiness — or you can accept it for what it is, even embrace it, because there's a difference between the two."

Jason Michaels: Wow, your Mother was very wise.

Dave Pittman: Accepting something says, "I have to do this thing." Embracing it says, "I get to." It's about realigning the position and attitude of your heart. For whatever reason, in God's sovereignty and His purposes, He's allowed me to have this. So I can either be miserable or embrace it for what it is and trust that He has some other plan that I can't see right now.

Mom used different examples in the Bible to make this ring true for me. A major one that sticks in my mind was about Paul, the apostle who had a thorn in his flesh. In 2 Corinthians, speaking to Paul's affliction, God says, "My grace is sufficient for you."

Paul asked the Lord three times to take it away and God's answer was, "My grace is sufficient for you, and my power is made known through your weakness." For whatever reason that stuck with me. It was God.

When mom relayed that story to me, I'm like, ***Okay, I may not understand why God allowed me to have this, but if His power is made known through my weakness, I'm happy to bear it and embrace it for His glory***. From there on out, I was like, ***Man, I can do this.*** It just lit a fire underneath me to become more comfortable in my own skin and with my Tourette's. More importantly, I realized that my identity wasn't in Tourette's.

My identity was in Christ and Christ alone, depending on who He said I was. All of that to say, I finished up fifth grade with a newfound confidence in myself rooted in my Christ identity. This transformation made my entire family comfortable enough to put me back in public school in a different district. So, I went a hop, skip, and jump over to a new neighborhood, and that sixth-grade year, things really began to change for me.

The fear had been rooted in telling people about my condition. If I did, I was scared it would make me feel worse. However, what I didn't understand was that talking about it freed me from my condition's control.

I'm sure my peers were like, ***What is he doing and why?*** My parents decided to be proactive and make a video that explained Tourette's, which we then shared with the students, staff, and faculty. It explained all the details of my condition and that it wasn't contagious. I was worried that letting the cat out of the bag would lead to being made fun of more. Yet it actually did the opposite, and the teasing stopped. The kids were like, "Oh yeah, that's cool, that's part of Dave. He has Tourette's, no big deal."

Jason Michaels: How did this change you?

Dave Pittman: It was eye-opening. I could have stayed in the dark, held it in, and felt like a slave to the Tourette's. Or, I had the choice to let it all out and be open and honest with others. Fortunately, I chose the latter, and the bullying and mocking stopped.

That decision opened so many pathways for me. Not only was it healing for the past, but also for the future in terms of where life was going to take me. From that moment forward, I was headed down a journey that I couldn't yet see.

Thanks to being comfortable in my own skin, I stopped taking medication. I know that some people need it because their tics are far more severe, but I opted not to take it. I was like, "This is me, take it or leave it," and I actually functioned better without it.

Jason Michaels: Did that sudden surge of confidence carry on into adulthood?

Dave Pittman: I graduated high school and had no plans to go to college afterwards. I spent four years trying to figure it out. I was working three jobs — and basically homeless. Actually, I had an apartment, but the water was shut off a few times. I would go to the local

Holiday Inn Express, into the lobby bathroom just past the desk, with a duffel bag to clean up the best that I could. I reached the end of my rope, the end of myself, and finally surrendered my life completely to God. I was like, ***God, whatever you want from me, I'm all yours.***

About a week later, my dad called me and said, "We've got this opportunity. You might have to go to college in order to get it." I was like, "What are you talking about?" He said, "A group from Liberty University and their director just came down." As a side, my dad is a worship pastor in Arkansas at the church I grew up in. Specifically, he is a music pastor and had a group visit from Liberty University to do a concert. He'd had the privilege of taking the musicians out to dinner after the concert where he talked about life and what his kids were doing. My dad also told the group about my singing abilities, but that I, unfortunately, wasn't happy with where I was in life. The director said, "You should have him audition for one of the ministry teams. The auditions end in the next two weeks. In fact, don't even send the audition CD to the school because, if you do that, it won't get here in time. Send it to my personal address."

So, I went back home to lay down this audition track, which consisted of a few songs, and then sent it out. About two weeks later, the director calls and leaves a message on my mom and dad's answering machine saying, "Hey, Mr. Pittman, your son's quite good. I'd love to talk with him further about being the lead singer for a new male trio that we're putting together."

He was putting this new male trio group together as a part of one of the teams under the Department of Ministry. The best part was he wanted me as one of the male vocalists. Out of 1,000 guys or so who had applied, they picked me for the lead singer; and it came with a full tuition scholarship to a private Christian university.

Also, remember that I had no plan prior to this miracle. School was always difficult, so I had no plans to go to college. I didn't like traditional educational systems. But it's funny how God works because He will sometimes stretch you out of your comfort zone. He knows exactly how to get you onto His path. So I was like, ***I love music; I love singing; and then there's school.*** I knew I couldn't have one without the other, so I had to do this thing.

After weighing my options, my response was, "Okay, let's do it." Dad makes the call to the director and confirms. From there, I made the trek to Liberty University where I spent four years traveling and touring with the group, as well as being a full-time college student. However, it took me some time to figure out my major as what I originally declared, business management, wasn't for me. I knew that I'd be on the road at some point and would need business acumen but took one semester of microeconomics and was like, *Nope!* I think, probably, it was more the professor that turned me off to the subject than anything else. If I had stuck it out, it probably would've been okay, but that's not the way the story goes. So I changed my major to religion, which is what I earned my degree in when I graduated in 2008. The goal was to continue to pursue my music career, or "music ministry" work as I called it.

After school ended, I temporarily left all my stuff in Lynchburg, Virginia where Liberty is located. Next, I went home to audition for a few Branson, Missouri shows. While some of them seemed promising, they never panned out. Around the summer of 2009, my dad asked me one day, "Have you ever thought about trying out for American Idol?" My rapid response was like, "Of course!" I had watched the show throughout the seasons but was never able to audition because of either work or school.

Yet, I was free at this point with nothing to hold me back. So I said, "Hey, let's do this!" I drove seven and a half hours down to Dallas, Texas to audition in Arlington Stadium, also known as Cowboy Stadium. We were the first event ever to be held there. It was brand new.

Jason Michaels: That's a cool place.

Dave Pittman: The Cowboys hadn't even played there yet.

Jason Michaels: That's awesome.

Dave Pittman: The first round was called "the road auditions," and even with 11,000 strong there in Dallas, I made it through the masses. I slept on the concrete in between tryouts like you see others doing on the show and made it through the first round. After I came back several times over a three-month period, I ultimately made it to the big time: Hollywood.

Jason Michaels: What was that like coming from a relatively polar opposite environment?

Dave Pittman: During Hollywood Week, I made it to the Top 70 but was cut during the filming of the show. After my "American Idol" career ended, I moved to Nashville to further my career, where I stayed for nine years. During my time there, I put out two albums. The first one was "Crazy Brave," and the second was "A Different Kind of Love." After those releases, we toured for about a year and a half until my wife and I decided it was time to move back to our hometown in Arkansas.

Jason Michaels: In your bio you mention that your focus is spreading hope and love to the world. Why are you so focused on sharing hope with others? How has this powerful force for good helped you to manifest a better life despite having Tourette's?

Dave Pittman: I understand and know my identity comes from God. I am who He says I am through Christ's actions. Despite the difficulty, suffering, or pain we may go through in life, our personal relationship with Jesus provides hope. This may not be what the world defines as "hope." Rather, in the family of God and body of Christ, we know who we are and who we belong to. Hope has nothing to do with earth because it is eternal in Heaven. I wish for others to know this kind of hope so they can spend eternity in Heaven with Christ. It is possible for them to have peace and joy, rather than doom, gloom, and hopelessness, which the world constantly projects.

Jason Michaels: Okay, let's just say somebody's looking at this and they're mad at God. Why should they reconcile that anger and want a relationship with The Creator who gave them such a difficult existence? It's easy to understand a mindset that says, "I'm mad because this life is very difficult."

Dave Pittman: I don't think there's anything wrong with not understanding or even being upset at God, within reason, for His decisions. We see a lot of examples of this in God's word.

For example, take Job. If you have read Genesis, you know that Job questioned God. Job suffered. If you've read of Job's misfortunes, you know they stemmed from God taking away his family, money, and possessions. All that suffering was allowed by God. Yet Job didn't denounce God because he knew that he was His servant. He loved God and trusted Him no matter what He allowed to happen. No matter what, Job trusted Him at the very end. Still, in spite of his faith, he finds himself asking, "Why are you doing this? I'm innocent, test me, find me innocent because you know that." At the end of the day, though, he still accepted his lot. He embraced what he had, trusted the Lord; and at the end of the story, God restores all things lost back to him. He comes through for Job.

Jason Michaels: Have you seen your faith in God demonstrated even when it seemed that things were falling apart?

Dave Pittman: God chooses what He does for His glory and for our good. That means we must surrender what we can't control to Him, because if we could, then we'd be our own God. God may have some better purpose or plan that you can't see that second. However, He'll eventually open your eyes so that you can understand His actions. My own prayer became, "God, I surrender what I don't understand in the moment," so I could willingly turn my trust over to Him.

It's interesting to see, looking back now, how God's hand was always at work in my life. I couldn't see as a nine-year-old that he would one day use my brokenness to bring other people hope. As humans, I believe we are all broken and carrying Adam's sin from way back in the Garden of Eden. We are simply born with this burden. Fortunately, Jesus Christ is our Savior since he died on the cross for our sins. He took on our sins, ensured that we knew Him, and restored the broken relationship between His creation and the Creator.

Jason Michaels: To your point, since none of us can predict the future, something permanent like suicide, which you thought about as a kid, is never acceptable. We must trust in God's plan and know that he is using us as a force for good as his instrument.

Dave Pittman: That kind of finality is basically saying that God doesn't know what He's doing. That kind of action says that you, yourself, are wiser and know more than your Creator. Clearly, you don't. God has His purposes and plans, which are sometimes a mystery.

Jason Michaels: He uses the broken people as it says in the Bible.

Dave Pittman: People who have a speech impediment, such as Moses. You've got the fearful ones like Gideon in the Old Testament, who God fights a battle through. He uses Paul, who formerly persecuted Christians in the New Testament, and converts him on the road to Damascus. God used Paul even though he [Paul] spat upon His face. Those Biblical stories are just a few examples of the hope and love I want people to know as I have. God has purposes and plans for your life that you can't see yet. The only way to know that hope is through a personal relationship with Christ.

Jason Michaels: So, as someone who was bullied terribly in fourth grade, what would you say to a teacher who might read this and be dealing with similar situations in the classroom? Is there a way that they can support someone with Tourette's?

Dave Pittman: Most important is being present and aware of what is happening in all dimensions of your students' lives. It is important to also peek into their home life, even though I know that's such a fine line these days. Keeping a look out for how young people and their peers interact with one another is important. When it comes to Tourette's, there is no hiding this condition. Tourette's issues are generally visible, which is helpful. However, it is still key for a teacher to use their intuition. They need to be aware of what is going on in that student's life and really listen to what they are saying. Be authoritative, provide guidance, and show you really care by listening.

Like everyone, I had some teachers who were not invested. They simply showed up, taught, and then went home. Rather than a teacher, they were there to perform a job. The good ones always had my best interest at heart. They wanted to help me succeed despite what I was going through physically, emotionally, or spiritually. Whatever it took, they were willing to do it. My advice for teachers is to look at your work as more than a paycheck. Really seek to understand your students' hearts, lives, and personal situations.

Jason Michaels: A lot of people might imagine that a condition such as Tourette's could hinder your success. After all, the music business is a very difficult one to begin with, even if you are in perfect health. Is there any benefit of Tourette's that you can point to which has helped you pursue life and all that you're passionate about?

Dave Pittman: Honestly, I think being comfortable with who I am has been the greatest reward of Tourette's. Identity is about being at ease in your own skin. A condition or disability should never infringe upon this or stop you from living as a normal human being. Sure, there are setbacks to certain conditions like Tourette's, but that is just life, period. You have to swallow them and just keep going. We all get knocked down, but you don't stay there. We persevere through even the hardships and suffering. The key factor is to remember to let go of control over what you can't control.

Jason Michaels: What is a blessing that you've been given thanks to living with Tourette Syndrome.

Dave Pittman: I can clearly see the way God has worked for my good. Tourette's is the platform God uses. Music and singing are the vehicles. Both of those mediums are how God has gotten me to where I am today. He is at the source of everything. God's done it all. I give [Him] all the credit, and any success I've had has been Him and Him alone. God has been there throughout my journey to lead me where I am today. Ultimately, every action was for His glory — using Tourette's as the primary platform for His messages — and music as the vehicle.

JASON'S SUMMARY

The central theme to what Dave chose to share with us in his interview is his faith in God. Through numerous examples, Dave refers to the relationship that he has with his Creator.

The simple fact is that faith and resilience work together. While faith in God isn't required to become more resilient, those with faith in a higher power view the world from a different perspective.

One of the passages that stuck with me was when Dave stated, "I just remember Mom and Dad drilling into my head, into my heart, the importance of accepting yourself for who you are. As a believer, they showed me that what truly mattered wasn't just who I was in the world — but rather who I was in Jesus Christ."

Dave then further defines his character as, "I realized that my identity wasn't in Tourette's. My identity was in Christ and Christ alone, depending on who He said I was."

I have often stated that while I may have Tourette's, it is not who I am. In fact, one of my favorite exercises when I work with groups who want to increase their resiliency is to have them make a list of all the personality traits, interests, and passions they can think of that make each of them up. By doing this simple exercise, and then taking a good hard look at each of these factors, we can see that Tourette's is just one small part of a very complex individual. There is perspective indeed when you zoom out and look at things from a 360-degree angle.

I was also moved by Dave's desire to bring "a bit of hope to the world." While people of faith do not have ownership over spreading this message, they do often possess the desire. I would encourage anyone who feels compelled to lift others up, to pursue this calling. Because he responded to his calling, Dave has touched millions through his music.

Dave's comment about being "headed down a journey that I couldn't yet see," also struck a chord because it is yet another example of perspective. When I speak to groups about overcoming challenges and obstacles, I always include how important looking at the bigger picture is in that process.

The final thing that really stuck out to me in Dave's interview was when his mom defined the difference between "accepting" that he had Tourette's versus "embracing" it. What a major milestone it was when Dave adopted that perspective, because it elevated him from victim status to one in which he could leverage all that Tourette's had to offer. If that happened to get by you, I encourage you to go back and read it one more time whether you have Tourette's or not. Embracing a challenge, instead of merely accepting it, is a major shift in mindset that we should all strive to achieve.

To watch the video of the full interview with Dave Pittman, access additional tools to help you live and thrive with Tourette Syndrome, and connect with the Tourette Warrior community, please visit TouretteWarrior.com

ABOUT TOURETTE WARRIOR

I hope this book has inspired you and helped you realize that there are many people with Tourette Syndrome who are living successful lives.

The dreams that you have for your life as a Touretter are completely attainable. While your goals may not be attained overnight, by showing you other high-achieving Touretters, I hope to encourage you to make your own dreams and goals a reality. That is why I wanted to share the stories of all the incredible people in this book.

One of the things I've learned since I became an author is that people consume information and learn through different mediums. I've also come to understand that there are a lot of people who don't enjoy reading or find it difficult to do. If this applies to you, I encourage you to watch the videos on my website. Listening to the interviews can be very beneficial as you can witness the subject's body language, tone of voice, and emotions through the screen. In addition to the individuals featured in this book, I will be uploading future interviews with other successful Touretters. My goal is to keep adding video interviews to this website to inspire my community.

As part of the website, I am also including guided meditations designed to help you gain confidence, clarity, and more. Personally, when I meditate, my tics calm down, I am less emotionally reactive, and I feel more balanced as a whole. My mindset is more stable and less at the whim of this busy, chaotic world.

Finally, one of the greatest difficulties of living with Tourette's early on was a feeling of isolation. For many years, I thought I was the only one around me struggling with uncontrollable tics. Yet, listen up Friends, because there is no reason for you to ever feel like you're alone. That is exactly why I wanted to create this community of people living and dealing with Tourette's. This is where you can come and share your triumphs as well as your frustrations. Plus, you will always be cheered on because Tourette's is seen as a superpower, rather than a super curse. If you would like to join us on this journey, come be a part of our online community. The website where you can find video interviews, meditations, and a community of loyal supporters is below. Remember, Tourette Warriors stick together, so if you want what we have you know where to find us.

TouretteWarrior.com

ABOUT THE AUTHOR

Jason Michaels is an American magician, motivational speaker, two-time TEDx presenter, and author who lives with and thrives with Tourette Syndrome. Jason's primary goal with his programs is to amaze and inspire audiences around the world.

MAGICIAN:

Jason has shared his style of sleight-of-hand, illusion, and humor with corporate audiences, theaters, universities, the United States Armed Forces, and for private social affairs all over the world.

Jason's first full special, "The CardShark," can be enjoyed on YouTube. He has been featured on Penn & Teller: Fool Us, Stabal TV, Huckabee, JUDGED by Matt Walsh, in The New York Times, and in multiple industry magazines. Jason is the creator of the TV Pilot *Magician in the Kitchen*. He is also the star of "Jason Michaels Mobile Magic," the interactive magic show that happens on your phone on the Richcast app.

Additionally, Jason was the creator of the magic experience at Nashville's famed House of Cards and has entertained VIPs including Penn & Teller, Ambassador Mike Huckabee, Martina McBride, Kix Brooks, Jack White, Wynonna Judd, Brothers Osborne, Rodney Atkins, Dick Smothers, and more.

Jason is currently the International President-Elect of the International Brotherhood of Magicians. His show "Jason Michaels Live!" is available for bookings.

SPEAKER:

Diagnosed with Tourette Syndrome at age thirteen, Jason has overcome "the impossible" and become an internationally award-winning sleight-of-hand artist and professional speaker.

Jason is dedicated to motivating audiences to see beyond their challenges and self-imposed limitations with his keynote program #DOTHEIMPOSSIBLE: RESILIENCE. In this program, he teaches empowering techniques on how to overcome adversity and conquer the day.

In his follow-up keynote program #DOTHEIMPOSSIBLE: LIVE B-I-G, Jason inspires audiences to take action by living bigger, bolder lives by teaching the success and high-performance principles that made him an internationally award-winning entertainer.

Jason's newest keynote, MAKING MAGIC, blends sleight-of-hand and insights from the world of magic to help teams unlock creativity, elevate performance, and turn ordinary work into extraordinary results.

AUTHOR:

Jason is the author of the Amazon best-selling book "You Can Do the Impossible, Too!" His book details his "impossible" journey of overcoming the debilitating neurological disorder Tourette Syndrome to become a success in business and in life. This is Jason's second book.

THANK YOU!

Thank you for reading my book! I really appreciate your feedback, and I love hearing what you have to say. I need your input to make future versions better. Please leave me a helpful REVIEW on Amazon.

Thanks so much!!

Jason

RESOURCES/INDEX

Tourette Warrior Community
TouretteWarrior.com

Tourette Association of America
Tourette.org

Tourette's Action (U.K.)
Tourettes-action.org.uk

Tourette Association of Australia
Tourette.org.au

Jason Michaels Website
JasonMichaelsMagic.com

Nikki Burdine Website
NikkiBurdine.com

Jason Duika Website
JasonDuikaMotivationalSpeaker.com

Jacob Weiss Websites
HandEyeBody.com
PlayingByAir.com

David Shenton Website
ShentonMusic.com

Dave Pittman Website
DavePittmanLive.com

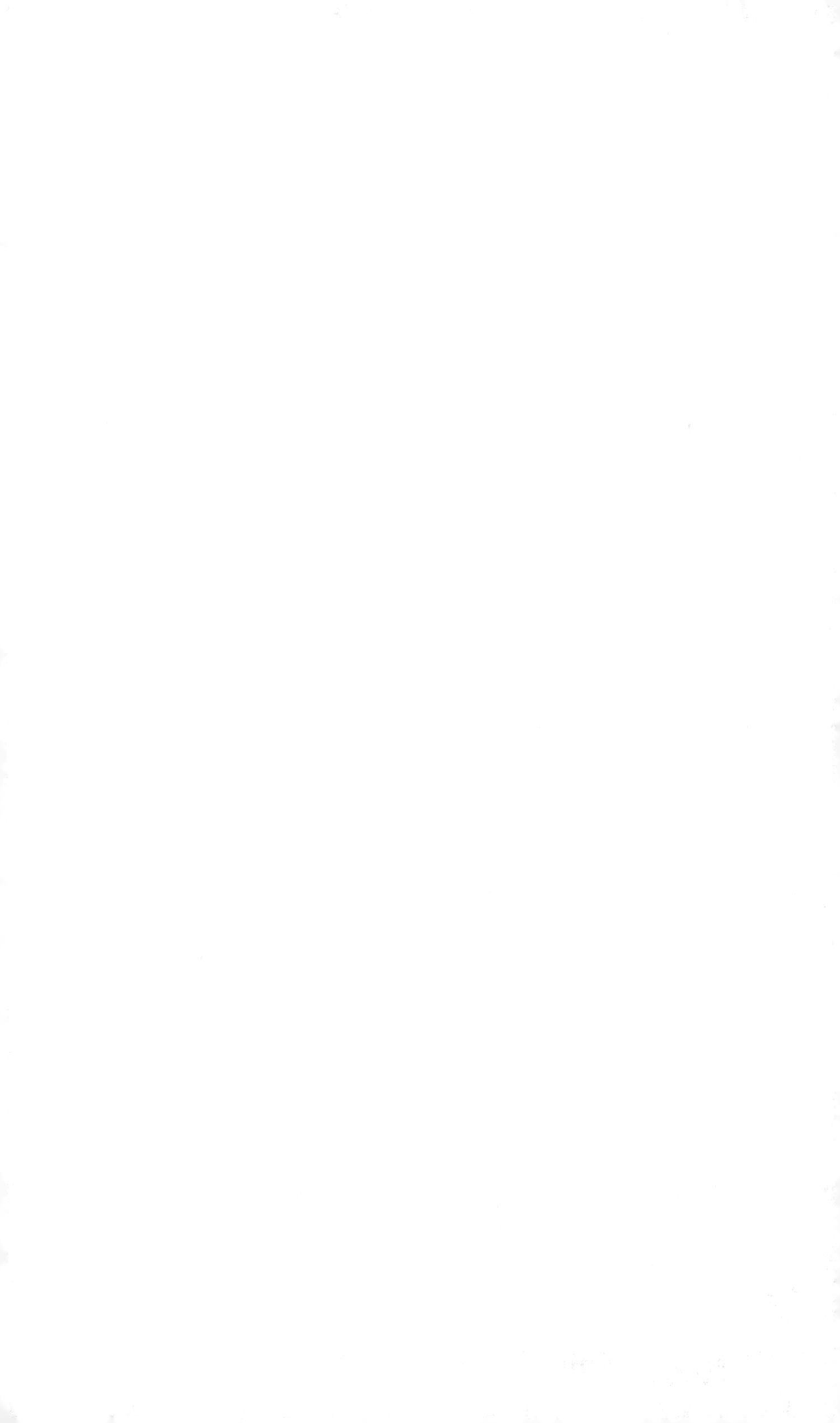

www.ingramcontent.com/pod-product-compliance
Lightning Source LLC
LaVergne TN
LVHW010702110826
845149LV00014B/3191

* 9 7 8 0 9 9 8 9 2 9 0 2 6 *